Nina McIntosh's

The
Educated
Heart

Professional Boundaries for
Massage Therapists and Bodyworkers

FOURTH
EDITION

Nina McIntosh's

The
Educated
Heart

Professional Boundaries for
Massage Therapists and Bodyworkers

Laura Allen

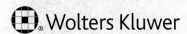
Wolters Kluwer

Philadelphia · Baltimore · New York · London
Buenos Aires · Hong Kong · Sydney · Tokyo

Acquisitions Editor: Jay Campbell
Product Development Editor: Linda G. Francis
Production Project Manager: Kim Cox
Marketing Manager: Leah Thomson
Design Coordinator: Stephen Druding
Artwork: Mari Gayatri Stein
Manufacturing Coordinator: Margie Orzech
Prepress Vendor: S4 Carlisle Publishing Services

4th edition

Trademarks and Service Marks

- Feldenkrais® is a registered service mark of The FELDENKRAIS GUILD®.
- The word Rolfing® is a registered service mark of the Rolf Institute® of Structural Integration.
- Trager® is a registered service mark of the Trager Institute.
- Rubenfeld Synergy Method® is a registered service mark of the Rubenfeld Synergy Center and Ilana Rubenfeld.
- Rosen Method® is a registered service mark of the Rosen Institute.

Library of Congress Cataloging-in-Publication Data
Names: McIntosh, Nina, author. | Allen, Laura (Massage therapist) author.
Title: Nina Mcintosh's the educated heart : professional boundaries for
    massage therapists and bodyworkers / Laura Allen.
Other titles: Educated heart
Description: Fourth edition. | Baltimore, Maryland : Lippincott Williams &
    Wilkins, [2017] | Revision of: Educated heart / Nina McIntosh. c2005.
Identifiers: LCCN 2016022648 | ISBN 9781496347312 (paperback)
Subjects: LCSH: Massage therapy—Practice. | BISAC: MEDICAL / Allied Health
    Services / Massage Therapy.
Classification: LCC RM722 .M37 2017 | DDC 615.8/22—dc23 LC record available at https://lccn.loc
    .gov/2016022648

RRS1606

Dedicated to the Memory of Nina McIntosh
(1943–2010)

I was very honored when Nina entrusted me with the future editions of this book. The third edition was completed while she was in a serious state of decline from amyotrophic lateral sclerosis (Lou Gehrig's disease). She always referred to this book as "my baby."

Nina started her professional career in 1970 as a psychiatric social worker in Denver, Colorado, after receiving a master's degree in social work from Tulane University. She soon became intrigued by the therapeutic possibilities of the touch therapies; in 1978, she trained as a massage therapist at what became the Boulder College of Massage Therapy. She became a certified Rolfer in 1981. Later, her interest in the psychological component of bodywork led her to study Rosen Method bodywork at Rosen Method Center Southwest in Santa Fe, New Mexico.

Nina's training in professional boundaries began in her social work graduate program, where physical contact with clients was thought to be so potentially intrusive and unsettling that students were prohibited from touching clients. As she began to practice bodywork, she saw that manual therapists, who routinely cross that powerful physical boundary, could benefit from knowing more about how to create safe environments for their clients and themselves.

Nina opened up the discussion about boundaries and safety with the first edition of The Educated Heart, *which became a standard text in many professional manual therapy programs. She also wrote a column on professional boundaries, "The Heart of Bodywork," that appeared in* Massage & Bodywork *magazine for more than a decade.*

In 2010, shortly before Nina's passing, she was awarded the Aunty Margaret Humanitarian Award at the World Massage Festival. She was unable to attend, and I picked up the award on her behalf. When I told her she was receiving it, she said, "I don't think I'm any kind of humanitarian," but she truly was. Her mission was to make the massage room a safe space for clients and practitioners. Her guidance has helped so many thousands of therapists to reach that goal.

Nina McIntosh was a friend, a role model, and a mentor to me. I'm honored to be taking care of "her baby."

—Laura Allen

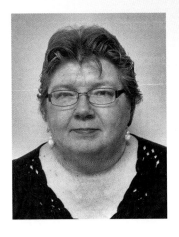 Laura Allen began studying bodywork in 1993, while still working in her career spanning more than 20 years as a chef and restaurant owner. In 1998, she sold her restaurant and accepted a job as the administrator of a massage school. A few days after taking the job, she decided that helping people feel better was the best job in the world, signed on for a weekend program at the school, and became a licensed massage therapist. Allen also returned to college at Shaw University for a degree in psychology, and detoured for 3 years to teach in public schools. She taught professional ethics and other classes at the massage school for 5 years, before leaving to open a multidisciplinary clinic in 2003.

Allen is the author of *One Year to a Successful Massage Therapy Practice* (LWW, 2008); *A Massage Therapist's Guide to Business* (LWW, 2011); *Clay & Pounds' Basic Clinical Massage Therapy: Integrating Anatomy & Treatment* (3rd ed., LWW, 2015); *Plain & Simple Guide to Therapeutic Massage & Bodywork Examinations* (3rd ed., LWW, 2016); several self-published books, and hundreds of blogs and magazine articles. A provider of continuing education since 2000, she has taught classes all over the United States, Canada, and the United Kingdom. In 2015, she accepted a position as the Massage Division Director of Soothing Touch, a family-owned massage and skin care product company located in New Mexico. In 2016, she closed her clinic to focus on that job, and continues to teach and write.

Allen resides in the mountains of Western North Carolina with her husband Champ, also a massage therapist, and their two rescue dogs.

REVIEWERS

Samantha Allen, LAc, MSOM, Dipl CH
Sandhills Community College
Pinehurst, North Carolina

Susie Byrd, MTI
The Edge School of Massage
Fayetteville, Arkansas

Fran Candelaria, MPH, BA, CMT
Brightwood College
Hammond, Indiana

Dawn Fortune-Brown, LMT, BCTMB
Nashville School of Massage Therapy
Nashville, Tennessee

Greg Hurd, LMT, MA Expressive Therapy
Bancroft School of Massage Therapy
Worcester, Massachusetts

Paula K. Jilanis, BCMT, MA, LMT
Allegany College of Maryland
Cumberland, Maryland

Steven Koehler, ND, BS, AAS, LMBT, CR, RMT, CMMP, CKTP
Program Chair/Instructor
Lenoir Community College
Kinston, North Carolina

PREFACE

This new fourth edition of *The Educated Heart* continues with the same engaging, insightful style and practical advice that is the legacy of Nina McIntosh, and is now continued by Laura Allen. The first edition was a pioneer in the field—the first book to focus solely on ethics and professional boundaries for the manual therapies. That edition was very well received by a profession that was realizing the importance of relationship skills in creating a safe and comfortable environment for both client and practitioner.

As did the previous editions, this new one continues the unique approach of the original *Educated Heart* with its conversational, nonjudgmental style, clear and easy-to-understand explanations of complex psychological dynamics, and real-life examples that bring dry concepts to life. We continue to offer practical suggestions for everyday boundary situations and sound advice for both beginning and experienced practitioners. Lighthearted cartoon illustrations of common scenarios give this sometimes anxiety-producing material a friendlier tone.

This new edition also features the greater clarity and organization of the third edition, making it easier to teach, and understand, with enhanced material on the dynamics of the client–practitioner relationship and specific suggestions for what to say to clients in common difficult situations.

The biggest change in this edition is the inclusion of the many boundary issues related to the Internet. The popularity of social media has had a huge impact on society in general, and there has never been a more obvious need for ethics education in this area.

Audience

This book is intended for all manual therapists or somatic practitioners, including massage therapists, bodyworkers, movement educators, practitioners of Eastern methods, and practitioners who work primarily with energy fields. Additionally, it addresses the professional needs of manual therapists in all phases of their careers and in any setting—whether private practice, a spa, a medical setting, or a massage therapy franchise. This new edition more comprehensively recognizes the diversity currently found in this profession—in specialties, practitioners, and work settings.

For students, it offers the support and information needed to establish the solid professional boundaries that will be important for their success and well-being. For experienced practitioners, many of whom were never schooled in the complexities of client–practitioner relationships, it provides the chance to learn new ideas to make their practices more fulfilling or to reinforce their own good decisions. Also, it is written so that readers need no prior knowledge of psychological concepts to understand the dynamics presented.

Scope

The Educated Heart was never intended to be a thorough discussion of every aspect of our work. For instance, although it offers good basic information on setting up a business and on working with clients who have been physically or sexually abused, these areas are not covered in detail. Some subjects addressed in this book, such as working with clients who have been abused, are probably best learned through in-person workshops that offer experiential exercises and more complete instruction. Readers will need to seek out such workshops to receive proper training in these areas while bearing in mind that no amount of workshops qualifies a massage therapist to act as a psychologist. Readers can also refer to the resources listed in the Appendix C: Related Readings for more information on topics that are not covered in depth. Note, too, that this book is not intended as a substitute for learning your local and state ethics regulations, the requirements of your professional associations, or any relevant licensing requirements.

Overview

Below is an overview of the main concepts and tools presented in each chapter:

- Chapter 1, "The Educated Heart: The Need for Professional Boundaries," covers why boundaries provide safety for both client and practitioner and why they are necessary in a professional relationship; it also presents seven major misconceptions about boundaries.
- Chapter 2, "Protective Circles: Boundaries and the Professional Relationship," discusses the concept of boundaries as protective circles that show both client and practitioner what is appropriate inside the therapeutic relationship and what is not.
- Chapter 3, "Framework: Nuts and Bolts of Boundaries," covers a wealth of nitty-gritty logistics and details of creating a professional environment, no matter whether you are self-employed or work for someone else.
- Chapter 4, "Client–Practitioner Dynamics: Boundaries and the Power Imbalance," discusses the concepts of transference and countertransference, including how transference creates a power difference that makes balance necessary and how countertransference can interfere with your compassion and objectivity.
- Chapter 5, "Ethical Boundaries: From Theory to Practice," presents guidelines for making ethical decisions, including how to make judgment calls in

ambiguous situations and tips on such issues as informed consent, scope of practice, and confidentiality.

- Chapter 6, "Boundaries and the Power of Words," gives general guidelines for effective professional communication with clients and specific suggestions for common situations that arise in various work settings.

- Chapter 7, "Sexual Boundaries: Protecting Our Clients," includes general concerns and specific help with maintaining appropriate sexual boundaries with clients, including clients who have been sexually abused or those who have a crush on their practitioners.

- Chapter 8, "Sexual Boundaries: Protecting Ourselves," deals with such issues as protecting ourselves from clients who make inappropriate sexual remarks, knowing what to say or do when a client has an erection, and dealing with sexual predators within the profession.

- Chapter 9, "Financial Boundaries: Getting Comfortable with Money" focuses primarily on suggestions for those who have a private practice or want to have one. However, if you wish to work for someone else, this chapter can be helpful in choosing an employer whose financial policies fit with yours. It covers general attitudes about money that might get in the way of success; how to create financial policies that you are comfortable with; and for those in private practice, the ins and outs of such issues as setting fees, charging for missed appointments, and giving refunds.

- Chapter 10, "Dual Relationships and Boundaries: Wearing Many Hats," presents different kinds of dual relationships, including working with friends and family, converting clients into friends, and doing trades or bartering, and how to avoid or minimize common pitfalls.

- Chapter 11, "Boundaries and the Internet," is a new chapter addressing the many ethical issues and challenges presented by the Internet and, especially, social media.

- Chapter 12, "Help with Boundaries: Support, Consultation, and Supervision," covers the need for getting outside help with client–practitioner dynamics as part of taking care of ourselves and different kinds of help and the advantages of each.

Key Features

The key learning features are listed below:

- Case examples, indicated by an arrowhead (➤), provide real-life scenarios of concepts and situations discussed in the text.
- Memorable quotes from the text are featured in the margins of each chapter.

- Key terms are boldfaced in the text and defined in the margins and in the glossary at the back of the book.
- Questions for Reflection help readers process and internalize the content presented in each chapter.

New in This Edition

Below is a list of new features and content in this edition:

- Consider This provides food for thought for making career-affecting choices.
- Real Experience, contributed by actual practitioners, shares problems and dilemmas that they've confronted in their own practices.
- More thorough discussion of the boundary problems faced by those who are employed by others—for those who work in spas, physicians' or chiropractors' offices, or for massage therapy businesses.
- As mentioned above, a new chapter (Chapter 11) on professional boundaries and the Internet.

Additional Resources

The following materials are available free at thePoint.lww.com/McIntosh4e:

- For both individual and classroom use, downloadable video clips both entertain and educate, depicting problematic boundary situations commonly experienced by bodyworkers and massage therapists. These will challenge students and practitioners alike to sharpen their responses.
- Instructors will have access to an Instructors' Manual that guides instructors every step of the way, beginning with:
  - Teaching Professional Boundaries, including why boundaries can't be taught by memorization, how to teach students the fun and easy way through interactive exercises and discussion, how adults learn best, teaching by example, creating a safe learning environment, dealing with students' emotional responses, guiding discussion groups, and taking the threat out of role-playing.
  - How to Use Suggested Lesson Plans—customizing lesson plans for your students; how to lengthen or shorten the course to fit your curriculum.
  - Chapter by chapter help—with general comments, key points, interactive learning aids, and sample tests, both essay and multiple choice
  - Related readings
  - Sample scripts for role-playing

- Test generator
- PowerPoint slides
- Lesson plans

Final Thoughts

In writing this book, it was my wish to help this profession find the public recognition it deserves. Quite simply, I think the key to that recognition lies in the quality of our day-to-day interactions with clients. Before the first edition, Nina McIntosh interviewed more than 50 experts in the profession about what makes a relationship healing. I have added to that with the Real Experiences contributed by working massage therapists and my own experience as a therapist and teacher of professional ethics for more than 16 years.

I have deleted very little of Nina's original text–only where it was timely to do so. Nina was not a big fan of the Internet, and was especially not a fan of social media, so the text has been expanded to include those now-important issues that were not covered in previous editions. I hope I have done well in leaving Nina's voice intact, and in not changing the "spirit" of the book at all, because it was and remains the singular most important book for massage therapists who are learning to deal with professional boundaries. The conclusion can be summed up in a few words: *Treat yourself and your client with kindness and respect.* For those of you who are interested in learning more about creating kind and respectful relationships, I hope this new edition will be a valuable resource and a useful friend.

Laura Allen

ACKNOWLEDGMENTS

First and foremost, I can never thank Nina McIntosh enough for being my friend and mentor, and for trusting me enough to hand over *The Educated Heart* to me. I miss her all the time.

I acknowledge my husband, Champ Allen, who goes months at a time seeing only the back of my head while I'm working on a book project and never complains.

Linda Francis has been my editor for more than a decade, and I'd never have had a word in print if not for her. She is always a joy to work with and guides me in the right direction without fail. I appreciate the whole team at WK/LWW for all they do for me.

I acknowledge Leslie Young of Associated Massage & Bodywork Professionals for being a dear friend to Nina McIntosh, and being so good to me, and I've always appreciated our little chats and shared remembrances of Nina, and the encouragement she has given to me.

I acknowledge the artist, Mari Gayatri Stein, for her contributions to this book. I know that Nina loved her, and I am glad that we continue to have her art in this book.

My undying gratitude to my mother, Margaret Lawson; my brothers Robert, Alan, and James Earwood; and Champ's sisters Sherry Allen, Penny Jones, and April Allen for their support. We were going through my husband's battle with Stage IV cancer, and an aneurysm that occurred just a few weeks after he finished his chemotherapy and radiation while I was working on this book, and their help and support was everything to us.

Finally, I have to acknowledge all the students who have attended my ethics classes for the past 16 years. They came to learn from me, but I've learned so much from them . . . the sharing that goes on in these classes is invaluable to everyone present, and I truly appreciate it.

CONTENTS

CHAPTER 1

The Educated Heart: The Need for Professional Boundaries

While the practice of massage has been around since antiquity, our profession is still young. In fact, there are many who argue that we're not yet at the level of a profession at all. While massage is now regulated in almost every state, very few state boards consider massage therapists to be health-care providers.

We are still exploring what it means to be a good **manual therapist**. We are learning that technical skill is only one aspect of a responsible and successful practice. For our work to be effective, we need solid professional therapeutic relationships with our clients. We create such relationships by knowing what belongs in our interactions with our clients and what doesn't. We need to know how to communicate clearly with clients (and even potential clients) in a way that is professional. Clients will appreciate our friendliness and warmth. But more than that, they need the security of sturdy professional boundaries—and as massage therapists, we also need them for ourselves.

Our work is unusually personal. Other than doctors and nurses, we are the only people who (legally) place our hands on unclothed people who are in a vulnerable position. Consider that a total stranger walks in our door, and just a few minutes later, he or she is partially or fully unclothed and on the table, while our fully clothed body is standing over him or her, and we're putting our hands on that person. It's a huge responsibility not to violate the trust that people place in us, by their very presence in our massage room.

To many people, what we do is unfamiliar, and the intimacy of the work may stir up deep emotional associations. We also have to overcome the massage parlor

Manual therapists:
Trained professionals who touch the body of the client or who use a method of movement to affect the body of a client for the purpose of facilitating awareness, health, and well-being. As used here, the term is interchangeable with somatic practitioners and includes massage therapists, bodyworkers, other health professionals such as chiropractors and osteopaths, movement educators, and practitioners of Eastern methods. While people who practice energy modalities are not truly manual therapists, in the context that they may not be touching the body, the relationship dynamics are similar.

imagery that has been associated with massage; there will always be sex workers who practice their trade hiding behind the word *massage*, since very few places allow the legal practice of prostitution. It's a potentially confusing and highly charged situation that we can only make safe for our clients and for ourselves by diligently maintaining professional boundaries and by practicing clear, direct communication with them about their own expectations and ours.

Attention to boundaries is also the key to a smoothly flowing work life. When we create a safe environment, our clients settle in and relax. We have more satisfied clients who come back and who tell their friends about us. When we respect the client's boundaries, we have fewer difficult clients and more clients who leave our treatment rooms with a lighter heart and a lighter step. When we safeguard our own boundaries, we protect our own emotional well-being and our own prosperity, leaving *us* with our own lighter heart and lighter step.

Most of us come to this work with good intentions and a genuine wish to serve others. These aspirations flourish best within the structure of good professional boundaries. To truly serve our clients, we need not just good hearts, but also educated hearts.

The Need for Educated Boundaries

When we hear the word "professional," we may think of a clinical atmosphere or a distant and aloof therapist. But professionalism doesn't mean acting stuffy or keeping our clients at arm's length (no pun intended). It simply means that when we're working, our focus is on our clients. We give them our full attention; we listen to them; we're sensitive to their vulnerability. Being professional is just an educated way of being kind.

Being professional is just an educated way of being kind.

Boundaries:
In this context, a boundary is like a protective circle around the professional relationship that separates what is appropriate within that relationship from what is not.

The best way we can demonstrate this kindness is by observing appropriate **boundaries**. Clients instinctively feel safer when we set clear boundaries. Maintaining good boundaries is also a kindness to practitioners. Not only do we feel more secure when expectations are clear, but also our work is less stressful and more rewarding.

Understanding the Need for Boundaries

Whether we work in a spa, a doctor's office, or on our own, our success depends, to a large extent, on how we handle our professional relationships. No matter how technically skilled we may be, our clients won't get the full benefits of our work if they don't feel secure with us. A casual attitude toward boundaries can jar clients and make them uneasy. When people complain about a manual therapy session they received, their complaint is not usually about the practitioner's inability to name all the muscles in the foot or inadequate effleurage. Instead, they'll say, "She talked about her divorce the whole hour" or "I felt nervous going to a bodyworker who works out of a bedroom in his house."

To understand why safe boundaries are crucial, we have to be aware of the special circumstances of our work, particularly the physical intimacy, the effects of touch, and the power dynamics in our relationships with clients.

Keeping Clients Safe

Much of the public does not have a clear idea of what we do, how we are trained, and what to expect from us. They may associate our work with the sexual overtones of massage parlors. They may be wary of our lack of traditional medical credentials or may fear that we will injure them or make a physical problem worse. They may have heard of a friend's experience with a barefoot massage therapist burning sage in the room and banging a gong to "clear the negative energy" before beginning the massage. It is up to us to make the situation a safe one in which they feel comfortable and where they can relax and heal. It is up to us to show that we are serious about what we do and that we are genuinely concerned about our clients' welfare. Maintaining appropriate professional boundaries is a crucial step in setting the right tone for safety. We have the obligation to *first do no harm*. That doesn't just mean observing contraindications for massage; it also means to honor the integrity of the therapeutic relationship.

For us, the intimacy of our work is something we can take for granted. It can be easy to forget how scary and potentially intrusive some clients may find physical touch—particularly those who have never experienced massage and don't know what to expect. We live in a culture in which touch is often experienced as leading to seduction or violence. For many people, something as ordinary as sitting in a waiting area with someone in the seat on either side of them, or accidentally brushing up against someone they don't know, is uncomfortable. Some of the people we see may have even been the victims of violent or sexual assault at some time in the past. Yet in our work, clients agree to be touched by a relative stranger usually while they are naked or only partially clothed. Some clients may have body-image issues and fear our negative judgments about their physical appearance. In a society obsessed with being trim and blemish free, clients are revealing their less-than-perfect bodies to us. No wonder some people have a hard time letting go.

Uncovered Feelings and Memories

Touch can bring up long-buried feelings and memories that clients may find surprising or even alarming. Even in the most caring of families, certain feelings or aspects of ourselves can meet with disapproval from those around us. As children, we unconsciously learn to hold back these feelings. We may also protect ourselves by blocking out unpleasant or traumatic memories. Without being conscious of it, we may hide uncomfortable experiences or emotions—perhaps even from ourselves.

When we hold back our feelings, aspects of ourselves, or memories, we may literally do so with our muscles. We grit our teeth or grind them in our sleep from stress, creating tension. We let that person we don't get along with at work, or some situation that makes us uncomfortable, become literally a pain in the neck from holding in stress and tension. This is true whether the stressor, and the subsequent holding pattern, began last week or decades ago. When clients are touched, especially as their muscles relax, those memories and feelings may emerge.

Sometimes the results are dramatic.

➤ *A 60-year-old client tells his massage therapist that he's never had any injuries. However, when his therapist works with his lower leg, memories come flooding back of falling out of a tree and spraining his ankle when he was 10 years old. As if it were yesterday, the client remembers how it happened, how his mother reacted, and how scared and hurt he felt.*

But more often, the tie between the muscle relaxing and the memory emerging may be so subtle that it goes unnoticed.

➤ *After her massage therapist loosens up her tight shoulder muscles, a client suddenly remembers an argument with her ex-boyfriend that ended in a breakup, and how angry she felt at the time.*

➤ *As her therapist works quietly and deeply, a client begins to cry, realizing how much grief she is feeling over the recent death of a friend.*

Such releases of feeling are normal and usually beneficial to the client. We don't need to be concerned about them or feel that we need to do anything more than to provide a sympathetic ear or a tissue. (If clients have tears, we might ask whether they want us to continue with the massage or give them a moment.) Clients bring their personal experiences, memories, biases, their stressors, and their own personality to the table—and we bring ours, without even thinking about it. Although many clients come to us basically for relaxation and can easily appreciate the simple pleasure of being touched without having such memories intrude, others who have experienced trauma may have a more difficult time letting themselves relax.

Most often, clients won't be consciously aware of suppressed feelings during the session; however, they may express those feelings in unconscious ways. For instance, a client who was physically or sexually abused may be wary of his or her practitioner or may cringe as a certain place on the body is touched, or expect to be harmed without knowing why. Even if potentially scary or unpleasant material doesn't emerge, our touch may nudge the edge of it. Veterans who are suffering from posttraumatic stress disorder (PTSD) due to war, people who may have lost a loved one recently and are in one of the stages of grief, a person who is being a care-giver for a sick family member, or someone who has just gone through an emotional upset may be in a more vulnerable state than another client who isn't experiencing any such thing. We can't judge by superficial appearances how emotionally fragile any one client might be. Because of that, we need to provide safe and reassuring boundaries for *all* our clients. In fact, it is *imperative* that we avoid doing anything more than providing a safe space and reassuring boundaries for clients. Unless you are a licensed psychologist, clinical social worker, or otherwise qualified in addition to being a licensed massage therapist, it is out of scope of practice to counsel clients or give them psychological advice. Some massage school programs or instructors, bodywork modalities, and continuing education providers actually *promote* facili-tating emotional release in clients, and having a few hours of education in working with emotionally distraught clients is just enough to delude some therapists into thinking it's okay to ignore scope of practice and ethical client boundaries. It is not—but it is important to be aware that an occasional client may experience an emotional release while on the table, and to be able to respond professionally and compassionately if it happens.

Acknowledging Power and Responsibility

Power differential:
A concept used to describe a professional relationship where one person is viewed to have more knowledge and authority than the other, such as the client–therapist relationship.

The dynamics of the client–practitioner rela-tionship are complex and often subtle; there is a **power differential** present in any therapeu-tic relationship. Our clients automatically give us more power than they would, for instance, if they met us socially instead of in a profes-sional capacity, especially in a client–therapist relationship that is intimate in nature. They are often looking to us to alleviate their physical discomfort or emotional stress, which puts them in a vulnerable and often dependent position. Consequently, our words and actions tend to carry more weight and authority for them. Even though they may not be conscious of it, we can become bigger in their eyes—more like a doctor or parent figure. Clients may put us on a pedestal, thinking we can do no wrong. As practitioners, our re-lationship with clients brings with it built-in authority and responsibilities. Our task is to meet our clients' vulnerability with respect and kindness, and we do that by maintaining secure boundaries.

Seven Common Misconceptions about Boundaries

As much as we want to be respectful and kind, many somatic practitioners haven't been trained in either the whys or the ways of being professional. The dynamics of the professional relationship can be intricate, and the best course of action is not always clear. We may not even realize some of the mistakes that have arisen from our lack of education and awareness.

Some errors are more serious than others. Probably, no client will haul us into court for talking too much during the session about the movie we saw last night, but discussing a client's problems with an outsider could land us in front of an ethics committee. More serious offenses—including some that are unintentional—such as careless draping, or inappropriate comments or actions, could lead to loss of license, not to mention loss of reputation, lawsuit, or in some cases, criminal prosecution. Sometimes we can't gauge how big a problem our boundary mistake will be. The client who heard too much about last night's movie may not sue, but he or she may decide not to come back. Then again, he or she might be a longtime client who forgives the disruption of his or her relaxation—this time.

Some therapists have learned about the importance of good boundaries through painful experience—just ask anyone who has had to appear before a massage board to defend their actions or therapists who have grown resentful of their own practice because they have allowed clients to take advantage of their own lack of boundaries.

Some of us have had to piece together our own ideas of professional conduct without the benefit of specific training or education in that aspect of our practice.

Boundary Lessons

Years ago, I hired a young, fresh-out-of-school massage therapist as an independent contractor, and she told me during the interview she wanted to take Thursdays off. After several weeks, I noticed that she was always coming in on Thursdays, looking a little harried and aggravated (and not taking another day off to make up for it). When I asked her why she was there on her day off, the excuse was always the same: "That was the only day so-and-so could come." I advised her that was not true at all, and that by sticking to her guns and firmly saying "I am not in the office on Thursdays; let's see what other day we can get you in," she would see that the person would miraculously find another day to come. She didn't lose a single client over it—they did indeed find another day to come—and was free to enjoy her day off. It's good that she learned that lesson early in her career and is still thriving many years later, but if she had not stood up for herself early on, she'd probably still be allowing people to take advantage of her or totally burned out by now and gone from the profession altogether.

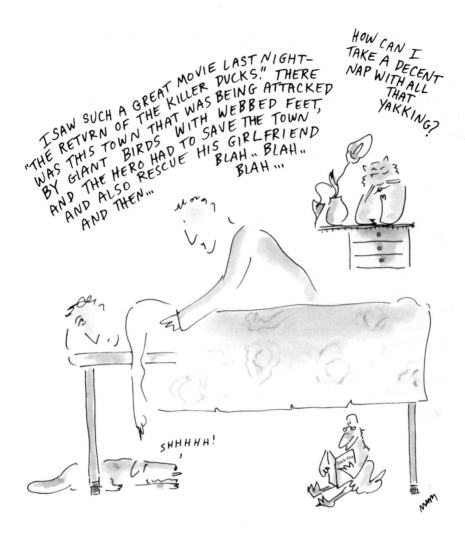

Education experiences vary; a huge number of therapists are not familiar with the laws of their own massage board. A student recently said to me, "My teacher didn't like ethics, so we usually spent the class talking about something else." As a result, some common misconceptions have been born out of understandable confusion. Clarifying these misconceptions can help remove any doubts about the importance of healthy professional boundaries.

Misconception #1: "I Want to Be Natural with Clients; Boundaries Create Barriers."

This concern about maintaining appropriate boundaries comes in many forms, such as "I want to be myself with my clients" and "I really want them to like me."

This is often how we justify talking about our own issues with clients or letting them see the off-duty side of us, confiding to them and complaining to them as if they were friends.

However, being professional means that we are careful about what we reveal to our clients, not out of a sense of superiority, but out of a wish to keep the focus on the client. When we share personal information with clients, especially our own problems, they may feel obligated to take care of us in the way that friends tend to do for each other. At the least, it takes attention away from the reason they are there—to have *us* pay attention to *their* needs. It's misguided to think that letting our hair down with clients is always therapeutic for them. When we are tempted to complain about our love lives, share our political beliefs, or tell clients how tired we are, we have to stop and wonder how that will add to their feelings of security.

It's true that some clients want to talk throughout the massage. It's *their* time, after all. Most people who chatter a lot usually just want someone to listen to them. Take your cues from the client. If the only words you are getting out of them are occasional grunts in answer to your asking them whether the pressure is alright, don't be a chatterbox. If they obviously want to talk, keep the conversation focused on them. Avoid conversation about controversial topics such as politics and religious beliefs. If the client brings up conversation that could lead to conflict or asks a personal question that you don't want to answer, the best response is "Let's focus on your body right now, so you can get the best benefit from your massage, " or a similar statement.

In rare instances, it can be helpful to let clients know that we too have struggled with the same kinds of issues. If we know a client well, we might want to reassure

REAL EXPERIENCE

During the very first massage I ever gave to someone other than a fellow student at massage school, the owner sent me into a session with an experienced therapist. She took her position at his head and sent me to the feet. As soon as I sat down, the other therapist started talking about her husband running around on her and her son getting arrested. I was mortified! I kept giving her little "shhh" expressions and giving her looks that said "SHUT UP," but she just kept talking. Even though I had only been in school a short time, I knew that wasn't the way it was supposed to go. I actually knew the man on the table, which made it all the more embarrassing to me. As soon as the client left, I was voicing my opinion to the therapist about how inappropriate she had been when the owner walked in, and she ended up getting reprimanded for her behavior.

—L.E.A., MT

or inspire him or her by remarking that we've faced the same problem, such as "I was diagnosed with fibromyalgia a few years ago, and I have found that exercising and getting massage regularly has really helped my symptoms. I go to the water aerobics class at the community college, and I try to schedule a massage every 2 weeks." However, such sharing should be carefully thought out. Unless clients already respect us and know our strength, talking about our struggles could make them question our capabilities, expect less of us, or feel obliged to help us. For the same reasons, we should mention only those issues that we have already resolved, and not bring up current problems, such as financial woes or relationship problems. Just as we should avoid giving clients personal advice, we should avoid asking them for it as well. This is especially true of clients who may be in the business of giving advice—counselors, ministers, clinical social workers, for example. Remember, they're on the table so you can take care of them—not to give you advice while paying you for the time.

The truth is that we do have more power in our relationships with clients; recognizing that fact is being responsible, not arrogant. But having good boundaries doesn't mean that we can't be genuinely caring people in our practices. Authenticity is reassuring and appropriate when we are down to earth in how we present ourselves and when we do not mystify what we are doing or pretend to be all-knowing. It can be healing to allow clients to see the compassion we feel toward them. We can, for instance, let clients see that their stories have touched us, and we can sympathize with them about *their* concerns, but it's not appropriate to ask them to do the same for us.

Boundaries aren't elitist or intended to make a client feel "less than" us or disrespected. It's quite the opposite; boundaries are a gift to clients.

Misconception #2: "I'll Just Use My Common Sense."

We may think that professional boundaries are just common sense, but it's not that simple. Making good judgments doesn't necessarily come naturally. Especially when a therapist is fresh out of school and hasn't had the time in practice to be faced with real-life ethical dilemmas, it's easy to make errors in judgment. After we've practiced long enough, we can begin to look and feel like naturals, but that's not the same as "just being ourselves" or only using common sense.

Without clear, thought-out guidelines, our decisions about boundaries and ethics are likely to be based on a hodgepodge of conflicting influences. We are affected by what our upbringing has taught us about pain, dependency, sex, and intimacy. We're swayed by our own perceptions, biases, and prejudices. Our judgment can be clouded by our egos and by the all-too-human need to be in control, feel like we're right, or feel important. Or, we may imitate mentors and teachers who themselves didn't understand the need for good boundaries and may not have been the best role model for how to behave. We may rely on advice from our friends or partners.

And when in doubt, we may throw in a random piece of wisdom from the latest self-help book we've read.

If, for instance, our own boundaries have been violated as children—sexually, emotionally, or physically— then what comes "naturally" to us may be off-kilter.

To make good judgment calls, we need to know ourselves well. Unless we are self-aware, our personal histories or trauma can interfere with making wise choices. If, for instance, our own boundaries have been violated as children—sexually, emotionally, or physically—then what comes "naturally" to us may be off-kilter.

We all have blind spots that interfere with our effectiveness. Even if we have had no significant childhood trauma, we bring to our work all of our personal history. We have rough patches in our behavior in which we do things that don't make sense or fail to see what's in front of us. We may deny, rationalize, and project the things we dislike about ourselves onto other people. Such failings are just human nature.

➤ *After gaining unwanted weight, a colleague found himself mentally judging his overweight clients. When he realized what he was doing and how it was related to his judgment about his own extra pounds, he was able to address and eventually change his negative feelings.*

➤ *A massage therapist with a history of being sexually abused by a relative routinely overlapped her social and professional lives, often urging people she found attractive to come to her for massage so that she could get to know them better. Until she sought professional help, she didn't realize the connection between how her abuser had overstepped family boundaries and how she was overstepping boundaries in her practice. Because being careless with boundaries felt familiar to her, she hadn't been aware that it was a problem.*

➤ *A massage therapist who had recently gotten out of a physically abusive marriage found that she was not able to massage males without feeling anger at her ex-spouse. After the manager pointed out to her that although her female clients raved about her, male clients rarely booked a second massage with her; she realized that she had made inappropriate comments about her ex-husband and men in general during sessions, and that her angry attitude had carried over to her male clients. She joined a support group for survivors of abuse, but soon left her job to open a mobile practice and limited her clients to women.*

None of us is perfect, but it's our responsibility to learn what professional boundaries are and maintain them. Good boundaries are too crucial to leave to just our common sense.

Misconception #3: "I've Learned Technique, and That's All I Need to Know."

Actually, your ability to maintain boundaries and to clearly and directly communicate with clients in a professional manner is every bit as important as your ability to give a good massage. Until recently, medical schools focused on teaching only anatomy and medical techniques, as if human relationships with patients don't matter. Perhaps, without thinking, we have used that same model in our profession. Many massage schools have stressed anatomy and technique, ignoring the importance of relationship dynamics. It's important that we realize that there's more to our work than physical mechanics. It's heartening to see that many massage and manual therapy schools (along with many medical schools) have added courses on boundaries, ethics, relationship dynamics, and the importance of a healing alliance between practitioner and client. It's hoped that we're moving past the idea that a client is simply a mass of muscles to be manipulated.

As manual therapists, we may need to pay even more attention to boundaries than doctors do. People don't expect to be able to let go and have a blissful, transcendent experience when they see their physician. But when people come to us (even if we work in a doctor's office), they hope to be able to relax and drop their defenses. They want to leave feeling not only physically better, but also more centered, more alive, and more themselves. To set the stage for that experience, we need a good deal more education and training than just learning the name of the erector spinae, for example. No technique, no matter how state-of-the-art it is, can ensure that a client will trust us. (Impeccable boundaries will not ensure trust either, but they will improve the odds.)

How people heal is a mystery. Humans are a complicated mix of psyche, spirit, body, and emotions, and we can't really know where one of these elements stops and another begins. We can learn a hundred new techniques and still not understand why people hurt. But we can create an atmosphere within which healing can take place.

Misconception #4: "I Don't Need to Know Anything about Psychological Dynamics; I'm Not a Psychotherapist."

Some of us feel it's not our business to try to understand our relationships with our clients. Perhaps, we fear that it will lead to "playing psychologist" with clients or trying to analyze them.

We're right to avoid analyzing clients' psychological problems, which is not within our scope of practice, and airing our opinions—that would be intrusive and a violation of boundaries. However, it is very much our business to learn how to create a safe emotional environment for our clients. And we can do that without inappropriately dabbling in psychological counseling.

All health-care professionals could probably benefit from knowing more about their relationships with clients. Only by understanding the more hidden dimensions

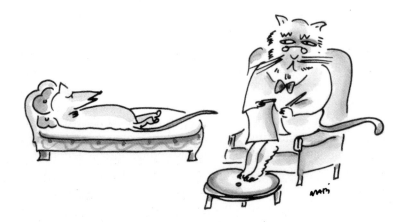

of the client–practitioner relationship can we have a deeper appreciation for the vulnerability of clients and their need for safety. We don't have to be psychotherapists to want to be sensitive to our clients' needs.

Misconception #5: "I Have Needs, Too."

A massage therapist who canceled a session at the last minute to attend to minor personal business didn't appreciate why her client was so upset. The therapist said, "My clients have to understand that I have needs, too."

Of course that massage therapist has personal needs—we all do. But there is a difference between *wants* and *needs*, and it's inappropriate to allow those *wants* to interfere with our work. We're there to focus on our clients' needs, which means putting our personal lives aside at times. Although we cannot avoid the occasional intrusion of an emergency or a personal situation into our work, we have to realize that being *professional* means that the show must go on, and when it cannot, we let our clients down. (We can consider offering a free or discounted session when we are forced to cancel without the standard 24-hour notice.) For example, rescheduling a client because you've come down with the flu is protecting the client; you don't want to make anyone sick. But rescheduling a client at the last minute because you just found out there's a one-day sale on at your favorite store or because you got a lunch invitation from someone you've been wanting to go out with is not acceptable.

We all have practical business we need to handle. It's a good idea to arrange your schedule, if at all possible, to have a regular day or half-day off during the week in order to be able to handle dentist appointments, going to the license plate office, or the other chores of daily living that must be done during business hours so that you don't end up canceling appointments to take care of those things.

At the same time, it's perfectly fine, and even desirable, to be concerned with our professional needs. We should ask our clients—or our employers—to treat us as

CONSIDER THIS

Most people seeking employment expect to be interviewed, and often fail to think that they should be asking important questions of the employer as well. For instance, what are their policies on cancellations and late arrivals? What are their policies on clients who make inappropriate sexual comments or gestures? You need to know that before you accept employment there. If you're self-employed, you're being proactive by deciding on your own policies before you open your business—and by informing clients of what those are. Clearly posting your policies on your website and brochures, having a sign in the waiting area, or giving clients an "Office Policies" sheet can help stop problems before they start. Here are some examples:

- Late arrivals will receive the allotted time left on their appointment. Full payment is expected.
- Arrivals that are more than 15 minutes late may be rescheduled at the discretion of the therapist.
- Cancellations with less than 24 hours' notice will be charged in full for the session.
- Anyone making inappropriate sexual comments or gestures will be dismissed immediately.

Remember, we're being kind to clients when we educate them about what we expect.

---

professionals and respect our professional boundaries. For instance, if we work for ourselves, we have the right to ask our clients to arrive on time, pay at each session, and give adequate cancellation notice. Ideally, we would want to work for an employer who upholds similar standards. If clients are allowed to take advantage of us, it can lead to resentment on our part and confusion on the part of the client.

Professional boundaries define the relationship as having limits and standards that both practitioner and client will honor. These standards benefit both parties by helping everyone feel more secure in what is a uniquely intimate situation.

Misconception #6: "My Connection with My Clients Is through the Healing Energy in My Hands, and That's What's Important."

Having "healing energy" is a vague enough term to begin with, and it's definitely not enough. Our work is intuitive, and sometimes our hands feel magically drawn to just the right place. We can have a subtle bond with our clients that is hard to define. But that isn't all there is to it. If we get too caught up in the mystery of our work, we can overlook our clients' basic needs. While you're working with your eyes closed thinking about the magical connection you have with the client, the client may be wondering why the room is so cold, why you were 10 minutes late, and why you keep forgetting his or her name. That's not being client-centered. Avoid the "I am the healer" syndrome, and keep your focus on the client.

Misconception #7: "But I Know Practitioners Who Are Careless about Boundaries and Still Are Successful."

In a certain respect, this statement isn't completely a misconception; most of us know someone like that. It's true that there are successful practitioners who disregard many professional standards and boundary concerns—maybe they frequently make friends with their clients, they're careless about confidentiality, or their treatment rooms are a mess. Most of these are well-meaning practitioners who never learned the importance of good boundaries. They benefit from the fact that clients will forgive a great deal if a practitioner has a good heart and "good hands." A careful look at their practices, however, generally reveals that they could make their clients much happier and their work lives much easier by paying closer attention to professional boundaries.

➤ *A successful practitioner gave a great massage but was chronically late in starting her sessions. As her clients waited on the table sometimes 5 or 10 minutes, they could hear her making phone calls or talking with her business partner. Although many of her clients were annoyed, few said anything. The practitioner noticed how hard she had to work to help her clients relax at the beginning of each massage, but she didn't realize how much her own behavior contributed to their tension. She just thought that all her clients were very uptight.*

Coming of Age

Good boundaries don't occur naturally. They need to be studied and practiced in the same way that we learn anatomy, physiology, or technique. The art of setting boundaries is the intangible element that brings out the best in both practitioner and client.

Although setting clear boundaries may, at first glance, seem to distance us from our clients, the opposite is actually true. Good boundaries don't create walls between client and practitioner; rather, they create a safe space within which we can touch clients' hearts and ease their spirits.

Questions for Reflection

1. In as much detail as you can, remember a particularly great massage you have had as a client or imagine what one would be like. What elements made it (would make it) a great experience? Are all of these elements related to the practitioner's knowledge of technique and anatomy? How many components are related to the professional atmosphere and the attitude and communication skills of the practitioner? Did they really listen while you told them why you were seeking a massage?

2. Have you ever personally experienced a release of feelings and memories during a bodywork session or a massage? If so, was it surprising to you that it happened? Did you feel that the therapist had an appropriate or inappropriate response?

3. Misconception #1 is about the concern that keeping professional boundaries leads to a less natural relationship with clients. Think about what has been true for you as a client or a patient. Has a health professional (doctor, chiropractor, massage therapist, or other bodyworker) ever been casual with you or self-revealing in a way that wasn't helpful or that affected your confidence in them? Has the opposite ever been true for you—that a health professional's behavior wasn't strictly professional, but you found it to be helpful? If you've experienced both of these, what made the one helpful and the other not?

4. As you were growing up, did you come to believe anything about pain, dependency, or intimacy that might interfere with your having a nonjudgmental attitude toward your clients? For instance, perhaps you were brought up to believe that only weaklings complain when they are hurt or allow other people to see their vulnerabilities. How would that belief affect your attitude toward clients who (appropriately) tell you about their aches and pains or share something about what is causing them stress? How might you unlearn attitudes that aren't useful to you as a manual therapist?

5. How easy is it for you to set limits? Do you tend to give in to extra requests from friends and family or business colleagues? Do you dread having to tell someone that you can't do something they want you to do? Conversely, do you find it easy to set limits but find that you can sound critical or harsh when you do so? Try to observe your limit-setting style, and, if necessary, find a way to practice setting limits kindly but firmly.

thePoint To learn more about the concepts discussed in this chapter, visit http://thePoint .lww.com/Allen-McIntosh4e

CHAPTER 2

Protective Circles: Boundaries and the Professional Relationship

Boundaries are like protective circles surrounding the professional relationship. Rather than being barriers that separate us from our clients, good boundaries safeguard both practitioner and client. Boundaries separate what is appropriate in professional relationships from what is not. When used well, boundaries clarify limits and expectations, helping to keep both client and practitioner secure.

In theory, the idea of staying within professional boundaries may sound simple. The client comes to us for massage therapy or bodywork. We do what we are trained to do and what we have contracted to do. The client pays an agreed-on amount or completes a prearranged trade. Although this may not sound complicated, it can be all too easy to lose our focus and overstep these boundaries. In understanding how to establish healthy boundaries, we first need to consider our role in the **therapeutic relationship**.

Therapeutic relationship:
A relationship between client and practitioner that is focused on the well-being of the client.

Understanding Our Professional Role

Taking on a role does not mean that we pretend; rather, it means that during our interactions with clients, we behave in ways that are appropriate to the **therapeutic contract**. The contract is determined by what we have been trained to do and, more importantly, by what the client is paying us to do. We may have training in clinical psychology, for instance, but if clients are coming to us for massage, we should not take on the role of psychological counselor.

Therapeutic contract:
An agreement between practitioner and client that is often implied rather than being explicit about what each will or will not do. An ethical contract must be within the bounds of the practitioner's training and the ethical standards of his or her profession. The client agrees to give specific fees, goods, or services in return and agrees to be respectful of the practitioner's guidelines for appropriate behavior.

We always have two roles with our clients: a specific role as a certain kind of somatic practitioner and a more general role as a professional. The first role—and the one most commonly recognized—is defined by our specific training, such as massage therapist, Certified Rolfer, or Trager practitioner. In this role, we use a certain method of massage therapy or bodywork to help a client. The broader role that we must learn is that of a professional person—that is the role that has been traditionally neglected and that can cause the most confusion. When we take on a professional role, for example, we need to keep our personal lives, opinions, and needs out of our sessions. Also, as part of that role, we expect to be treated as a professional with all that it entails. To have a solid and rewarding practice, every somatic practitioner needs to be comfortable in these two roles—both as a certain type of practitioner and as a professional. However, learning to be at ease with our roles takes time. We may be able to learn a couple of massage strokes in a weekend, but it takes a much longer time to develop a solid sense of ourselves as professional somatic practitioners.

The Professional Therapeutic Relationship: What Stays in

If boundaries form a protective circle around the professional therapeutic relationship, what is reasonable to include in that circle? The following sections give a brief description of the most basic elements of the professional therapeutic relationship, all of which are discussed more fully in later chapters.

Client-Centered Actions and Words

The concept of being "client centered" is central to the therapeutic relationship. Client centered means that our actions and words should be motivated by what is best for the client. Being client centered means that we put aside our personal egos, interests and needs, and likes and dislikes, and act in the best interests of the client. At the same time, this doesn't mean that "the customer is always right" or that we should let clients take advantage of us. After all, it's also in our clients' best interests to provide them with clear limits.

Being client centered means, for one thing, that clients have a right to ask for what they want. We don't want to become dictators, ordering clients to be quiet if we decide they're talking too much or becoming upset if they dare to ask us to vary our massage routine or adjust the pressure for their comfort. Clients need to be free to make requests as long as the requests are not abusive, destructive, or inappropriate. They should be encouraged to make their needs and wishes known. When clients do speak up, it's our job either to adjust and meet their needs or to explain why what they are requesting is not appropriate, in their best interests, or within the scope of our training or abilities.

Boundary Lessons

Therapists often overstep boundaries with clients, without even realizing they're doing it. It may come from a genuine desire to help someone, and still be wrong. We are supposed to do what the client has contracted for—and refrain from doing something just because it's our own desire, or because we think they need it. If a client states that he or she doesn't want a deep massage, but just wants a relaxation massage, imposing deep tissue work on him or her is not being client centered and not giving the client what he or she contracted for. If a client has not requested energy work, and you do that just because you want to do it, that is not being client centered and not giving the client what he or she contracted for. A new client once said to me that she had been to a therapist who hurt her during the massage, and I asked if she had spoken up and told the therapist that the pressure was too much. She stated that she had asked the therapist to lighten up, and the therapist responded with "I can't do that because this is what you really need." That's not being client centered in any way, and that therapist lost a client.

➤ *A practitioner complained about a client: "When I came back into the room after giving her time to get undressed and on the table, she had taken all the pillows in the room and arranged them around her on the table—under her knees and her neck and different places."*

In this story, one wonders why the therapist is complaining; it sounds as if the client is doing the practitioner's job for her. Unless the client was destroying property, there's no reason why she shouldn't make herself comfortable. We can't let our own control issues take over.

There are instances when we would not want to adjust to clients' wishes or automatically honor their requests. If the client's arrangement of pillows might interfere with the session in some way, the practitioner could always explain why the arrangement needs to be altered and ask the client's permission to make the change. Or, for instance, if a client has a pain in his or her neck and asks that we spend the whole hour working on his or her neck, we might want to suggest that because neck pain often reflects tension throughout the body, he or she might receive greater benefit from a more complete massage—but the bottom line is, unless it's harmful to the client, we should respect their wishes.

Confidentiality

If we want to be respected as professionals, we have to honor our clients' privacy and confidentiality. We cannot gossip about what they said, complain about what

Confidentiality is at the core of professional relationships. It begins with the first phone call and continues for the entirety of the relationship.

they did, brag about how much they liked our work, or in any way discuss or relate what clients said or did during our sessions (or during any professional contact). Confidentiality is at the core of professional relationships. It begins with the first phone call and continues for the entirety of the relationship.

A friend relates this breach of confidentiality:

➤ *I recently received a massage from a practitioner I hadn't been to before. I was surprised when she began telling me how one of her clients, a man we both knew, was responding well to her work. She talked about the physical problems he had had and what relief he'd gotten from her massage. I think I was supposed to be impressed by this report, but all it did was make me uncomfortable. I thought, "What will she say to other people about me?"*

If you work for someone else, a problem can arise if your employer doesn't enforce confidentiality. Here's how one massage therapist dealt with that issue:

➤ *After I began working in a spa, I discovered that it had the atmosphere of a gossipy beauty salon—both the owner and other massage therapists chatted casually about clients and repeated personal information clients had told them. I was tempted to join in, but I found that when I did, I didn't feel good about myself as a massage therapist. It also colored the way I felt about the clients when I saw them again because I felt guilty. Now I stay away from those discussions. I don't want to work in that atmosphere and am looking for a job in a more professional setting.*

Consistency

When asked what keeps clients coming back, many experienced therapists put consistency high on their list. Clients are reassured by consistency and reliability (assuming that we are consistently good about professional standards and not, for instance, consistently flaky or insensitive). After clients have gotten used to our settings and styles, they can be rattled by changes in routine, in the office space, in session times, and in any other part of our work with them. For instance, if a client has a regularly scheduled time slot, it's important to try to keep that time slot for him or her and not move him or her to a different time, if it's avoidable. If we do have to move our office or change a regular client's hour for good reason, we can be careful to keep other elements of our work the same. That doesn't mean you do the same exact routine every time; that will vary according to the client's circumstances

Breaches in confidentiality are running wild in massage therapy due to the Internet, and social media in particular. Hopefully, you don't post it on Facebook whenever you massage Mrs. Hoffman who attends your church, so why do some people think it's okay to post that they're massaging a celebrity? Every time the Super Bowl or some other big sporting event rolls around, Facebook posts start sprouting up: "I massaged Tom Brady yesterday!" or "Guess who I'm doing an outcall for? Venus and Serena Williams!"

The same happens with performers, artists, politicians, and other people in the public eye. If Christina Aguilera saw it on Facebook that she has a massage appointment scheduled with you, do you think she'd keep it? No, she would not. She'd look for another therapist who has the ability to be discrete. If a celebrity (or anyone else) posts on his or her own social media that he or she received a massage from you and it was great, that's not a problem. If he or she allowed you to take a selfie with him or her, then he or she has the expectation you're going to share that. Otherwise, keep your mouth shut about it.

Keeping confidentiality includes not only social media, but also avoiding privately telling friends and family, before or after the fact. People talk—including people who say "I won't tell anyone!" That's particularly magnified if you live in a small town. You may think it's innocent to excitedly tell your neighbor you have an appointment with a movie star—and the next thing you know, your parking lot is full of fans hoping for an autograph and a media frenzy waiting for them to exit the building! You'd better not risk that happening.

It is also a violation of confidentiality to mention people in a way that enables anyone with an Internet connection to find out who they are, even if you refrain from stating their name. For example, "I just massaged the CEO of Google!" or "I'm massaging the pitcher of the Yankees!" I've witnessed people who should know better, including massage school owners and instructors, doing this very thing. There is no gray area here; it is a blatant violation of professional ethics.

such as pain, injury or stress, and tension level. For example, if a client appreciates the fact that you use a lavender lotion, and all of a sudden you switch to something that's unscented, or vice versa, it could be stressful to him or her.

Of course, if we work for others, we don't always have control over when a client is booked, what lubricant is used, or even what therapy room we will use. Moreover, even practitioners who work for themselves have to make changes. (Helping clients adjust to changes is discussed further in the next chapter under "Sessions

Occur at the Same Time and Place at Regular Intervals.") Clients can trust us if we are professional and attentive to the details of their comfort, and they can relax more deeply if they can trust us.

Informed Consent and Right of Refusal

Informed consent may be withdrawn at any time, including after it has been given, whether verbally or in writing. If a client begins to feel uncomfortable with something you are doing, address it in the moment. They may feel nervous about telling you that they don't want you to touch a certain area, so be tuned in to body language and nonverbal clues. If they're flinching every time you touch a certain area, asking them if it's because that area is painful, or if they would prefer not to be touched in that area (and you don't have to know their reason), and adjust accordingly.

Informed consent:
It is a formal term meaning that clients have a right to understand all that is involved in our work with them, and we must have their educated, informed consent for our work with them to be ethical. It means that there should be no surprises for our clients.

There are also certain circumstances that may require more specific written, informed consent, and this is addressed in some, but not all, state board regulations. For example, performing lymphatic drainage on breast tissue, or performing pelvic floor work on clients. We have to keep in mind that many clients are ignorant of anatomy, and they don't *know* that the attachment of that sore leg muscle you're working on is in the pelvic area. Don't just surprise people by touching them in an intimate area; explain to them while you are at the insertion of their gracilis muscle where it originates (on the ischiopubic ramus, but you may say pubic bone to the client) and ask if you have permission to touch them there. There are a couple of states that allow massage therapists to perform internal work in body cavities (my state, North Carolina, is one of them). Specific written consent is required—and may still be withdrawn at any time.

As much as possible, we should spell out verbally and in writing our contracts with clients. They need to know what our training is, what methods we will be using, and the possible benefits and risks of those methods. We also have to let clients know that they can ask us to stop at any time and for any reason. They have what is formally called the **right of refusal**. It's never appropriate for us to be impatient or annoyed by clients who question our work or credentials or who don't want to take part in any aspect of our work. Clients need to know that we are offering our expertise but that they are ultimately in control of the session.

Right of refusal:
The right to refuse or withdraw informed consent to any aspect of treatment.

Our Rights As Professionals

Along with spelling out to clients what they can expect from our work and getting their consent, we need to be clear about what we expect of them. Upholding our

A massage-seeking client booked a session with a therapist he had never visited. He was escorted to the room and given instructions about being supine, and the therapist left the room. He was relaxing with his eyes closed when he heard the therapist reenter. After a few minutes, when the massage therapist had not yet touched him, he opened his eyes to see the therapist hovering over the table, with her arms sweeping back and forth over the client's body, and he asked what she was doing. "I'm clearing your negative energy," she replied. The therapist then proceeded to pick up a little gong and walk around the table several times banging on it. The client was incredulous but said nothing. After taking up about 10 minutes of the massage time with these ceremonies, the therapist finally got down to doing what the client had thought he was signing on for in the first place—a massage—and the next time, the client sought another therapist.

rights as professionals is an important basic principle for a healthy therapeutic relationship. We can, for instance, expect our clients to show up on time and leave when sessions are done. We can expect them to give us adequate cancellation notice and pay our fees on time. We should not work with abusive or disrespectful clients, and, indeed, we can decline to work with any client when we do not feel it is in our or their best interests to do so. (However, we need to be familiar with the codes of practice in our state or province that pertain to refusal to work with a client.) Also, those who wish to work for a spa or for another professional need to find out in the interview process their prospective employer's policies concerning the rights of massage therapists.

The Professional Therapeutic Relationship: What Stays Out

As somatic practitioners, we have to stay within the limits of our scope of practice, that is, the traditional knowledge base and standard practices of the profession. Staying inside those boundaries sometimes requires us to walk a fine line. Is it psychological counseling when we comfort a recently divorced client? Are we giving medical advice when we suggest that a client might not need his shoe lift anymore—one that was prescribed for him by an orthopedic doctor? Would it make a difference if it was prescribed by a chiropractor, or purchased over the counter at the drugstore? When are we crossing the lines of diagnosing or prescribing? When are we overstepping the line between friend and client? When are we giving too much personal information? If there is *any* doubt, that's a good sign you're about to cross the boundary line. Unfortunately, not everyone has the same ethical compass—which is why we have a code of ethics to point us in the right direction.

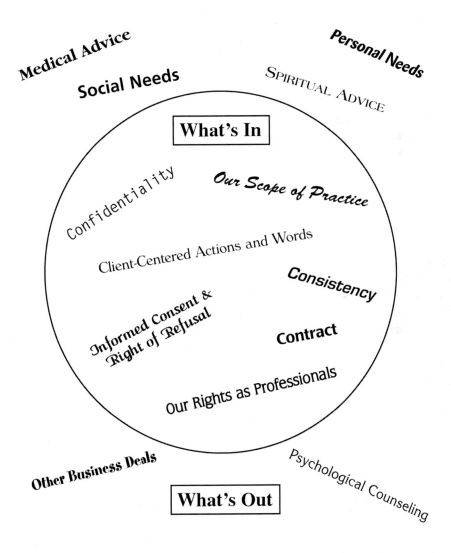

It's fair to assume that every somatic practitioner has violated boundaries, if only in some small way. Keeping good boundaries is a little like steering a car—it takes constant correction. Just when we think we're on a smooth path, we hit a bump. It's not a question of whether we make mistakes; we're human and we're bound to make mistakes. It's more a question of knowing when we've made mistakes and then being willing to change our behavior.

➤ *A colleague who often gave advice to an unhappily married client realized that he was in over his head. He told the client he would gladly continue to be a sympathetic ear for her, but if she wanted to work on changing her relationship with her husband, he would help her find a good marriage counselor.*

➤ *A bodyworker became aware that when he talked too much during a session, he literally would have a bad taste in his mouth. Now when he gets that taste, he knows it's time to be quiet.*

➤ *After a too-short vacation, a colleague realized she was dragging in just a few minutes late to all her sessions. As soon as she noticed this, she began making extra efforts to be on time and to take better care of herself.*

The challenge is to be aware of boundaries and value them, yet be tolerant of our own imperfection. However, because our mistakes are usually at the client's expense and can hurt our practices, we don't want to be too tolerant of our shortcomings.

There are three common ways that we venture outside the safe boundaries of the professional relationship: bringing in our social and personal needs, going outside our scope of practice and expertise, and mixing our work with other businesses. The following sections give a brief overview to highlight these major problem areas. All of these areas are discussed in more detail in later chapters.

Social and Personal Needs

Perhaps, the most frequent boundary confusion is between our professional and our social lives. Ways that we can overstep those boundaries range from the relatively harmless, such as an occasional lapse into too much chatting during a session, to the more problematic, such as socializing with clients and befriending clients, to the downright unethical, such as dating a client. Some of us don't understand why it's important to draw a boundary between our social and professional lives. What's wrong with sharing something personal about ourselves with our clients? What's wrong with a friendly cup of tea with a client? Maybe nothing is, but these actions might interfere with our professional relationships with our clients. Our boundary slipups usually have an innocent motivation. Some common reasons that we may want to bring our social needs into our professional lives are discussed in the following sections.

The Need for Social Interaction

Probably, the most common complaint clients have is about practitioners who talk too much. Clients are trying to relax and drift away into their own world, and we keep pulling them out of that world with our demands for their attention. Clients rarely ask us to be quiet. They won't say "I don't want to hear another word about your new boyfriend (your divorce, your new baby, or whatever it is)." Clients are both too polite and too influenced by the power imbalance inherent in the relationship. Rather than asking us to stop talking, they usually respond politely and then perhaps complain to their friends—or worse, not come back.

On the other hand, we don't want to have a rigid "no-chat" rule. Our main goal is for clients to trust us and feel comfortable working with us. In some instances, clients themselves have a need for social interaction with us. Here's an example from a colleague:

➤ *I work with a chiropractor who is warm, friendly, and very informal with his patients (whom he often refers to me). He has known many of these people for a very long time, and during his treatments he talks with these patients as you or I might talk with a coworker—sharing stories, information, or opinions about family, vacations, politics, and others.*

➤ *When I began working in his office, I tried to maintain a firmer professional and personal boundary, keeping my conversation with patients focused strictly on the work. This confused and baffled many of them, as they were accustomed to a more chatty level of interaction, and some of them misinterpreted my behavior as emotional distance, personal coldness, or a rejection of their desire to get to know me. In the end, I have chosen to adapt my style so that it more closely matches the doctor's. I still maintain a professional demeanor, honor patient confidentiality, and uphold ethics and standards of practice; at the same time, I have come to realize that every clinic or group practice has its own distinct dynamic, and there are many ways to express professionalism and maintain good boundaries.*

This is a great example of adjusting one's style for the sake of the client. The key here is that the therapist didn't lose sight of her professional role and her focus on the client's well-being. When you step outside boundaries, be careful that your aim is to meet the client's need for social interaction and not your own.

The Need for Friends

Some practitioners may say their clients are like friends. We may be on friendly terms with our clients, but are they really like our friends? Do we have friends who come to see us and immediately throw off their clothes and describe all their aches and pains?

There's a difference between a client and a friend. (And if our friend becomes our client, then the client role comes first during the session hour.) Personal friends put up with our lapses and our flaws; they listen patiently while we go on for 10 minutes about what somebody said to us and what we said back. They can let us know—and forgive us—when we hurt their feelings. Friends aren't paying us to be their friend—but we should respect the boundaries of the therapeutic relationship when a friend becomes a paying client.

As soon as someone becomes a client, we need to be aware of our therapeutic role, both in and out of sessions. The more we muddy the waters between the social and the professional, the more likely we are to do or say something that will interfere with having a professional, healing relationship.

➤ *A female bodyworker used a male client's sessions to lament the woes of her divorce and the problems of being single. This was confusing to the client—he wondered if she wanted a romantic relationship with him. When he asked her out on a date, however, she refused him. He felt hurt and rejected and stopped making appointments with her. This client ended up feeling wounded or betrayed by a relationship that should have been therapeutic. We usually cheat our clients when we put the focus on ourselves, when we ask them to listen to us and take care of us.*

The Need for Romance and Excitement

There's another reason to avoid the temptation to socialize with our clients. Let's be honest—when the wish to socialize is there, isn't it sometimes because we're attracted to that client? Or perhaps the client has a crush on us that we are enjoying. If we socialize with that client, what kind of message are we sending? Even if we are not flirting, the client may think we are. Because it's unethical to date clients or even to flirt with them, we'd be better off keeping the relationship strictly professional—and perhaps seeking some outside advice or discontinuing our work with a client for whom there is a strong attraction. The majority of state board rules address the issue of dating clients, even going so far as to spell out that you must terminate the professional relationship and wait x amount of time before pursuing a romantic relationship with someone.

Some of us can't avoid social interactions with clients. Those of us who live in small towns or are involved with small communities within a large town may have a difficult time keeping that boundary firm. We may frequently run into clients at outside events, friends and acquaintances may become clients, or clients may become friends. How to navigate these different relationships is discussed more fully in Chapter 10 on dual relationships.

Going Outside Our Scope of Practice or Expertise

We go outside boundaries when we make exaggerated claims about the effects of our methods or when we behave as if we are experts in areas in which we have either no training or only a relatively small amount of training. For instance, we are

REAL EXPERIENCE

I'm inserting my own real experience here because it's very relevant to this topic. In 2013 and 2014, I was hospitalized for serious illnesses (pneumonia both years; a urinary tract infection that went systemic into my bloodstream, and a diseased gall bladder). In late 2014, my husband was diagnosed with Stage IV cancer of the tonsils, which was further complicated by his life-long condition of chronic thrombocytopenia (extremely low platelet count). While I was ill, my husband posted updates about my condition on Facebook, and I posted updates about his condition, and our struggles in dealing with it, while he was undergoing the cancer treatment.

The out-of-scope, and in many cases, ridiculous and even harmful advice we received—95% of which came from massage therapists, was very distressing to me. I want to give people the benefit of a doubt, and believe that they have good intentions. However, when a massage therapist said *"Do not under any circumstances allow your husband to take chemotherapy!"* I was mortified to think that any client would forego medical treatment on the advice of a massage therapist!

Unfortunately, that incident was only one of many. We got advice to use essential oils, including swallowing them internally, from people who have no training other than the packet of sales pitches they got from their multilevel marketing company. We got advice to take colloidal silver, use clay baths, take the same clay internally, and make appointments with people who were holding themselves out as all manner of healers, among other things. I also received over 100 solicitations from massage therapists who were selling something. When I gave a simple "No, thanks" to one massage therapist regarding the (overpriced) supplement she was urging me to buy, she responded with "Well, okay, if you really don't want to help your husband." If she had been standing within my reach when she said that, I would probably have gotten arrested for aggravated assault. There is zero integrity in that kind of behavior, and I have no doubts that if they are acting this way with me, they are acting this way with clients. Such behavior is unethical, unprofessional, and does not belong in a therapeutic relationship. I feel sorry for—and fear for—the clients who see these massage therapists.

on thin ice if we guarantee that massage will lower a client's cholesterol level. Likewise, if we tell clients what foods to eat or why they should divorce their spouses, we have ventured into territory for which we have neither training nor contract.

Perhaps, the wish to inflate our work comes from the general insecurity of the profession. We don't live in a culture where ads on the bus read, "Got aches and pains?

Consult your bodyworker first." The benefits of massage are becoming more widely known, but many people still don't know how it can help them. For the most part, manual therapies are relatively unacknowledged by a culture accustomed to a traditional medical viewpoint. For many of us, there is a vast gap between what we know to be the value of our work and the value given to it by much of the public. Perhaps in our frustration with the lack of recognition, we swing the other way and promise too much.

Bragging, promising too much, and inflating the merits of our brand of work are all signs of insecurity . . . So is being insulting about the massage therapist up the street from you because she practices relaxation massage, while you perceive yourself to be superior to her because you specialize in deep tissue work. Our motivations for becoming somatic practitioners are complex, but generally, we have a desire to help people feel better. It can be difficult to tell them the simple truth—to say to someone who is in pain, for instance, "I can't promise this is going to get rid of your problem. You might even feel sore for a few days before you start to feel better." It may be harder to say, "I don't have enough training (or skill) to help you. Let me refer you to a more advanced practitioner (or another kind of health professional)." Sometimes, it is even necessary to say "I don't think massage is appropriate for you due to your medical history (contraindications, current illness, current or recent medical treatment)." But all professionals, no matter how advanced their skills and knowledge, need to know their limits—and stick to them.

The Weekend Workshop Syndrome

Many of us are constantly looking for ways to advance our knowledge of ourselves and our work. We go to workshops to add new techniques to our repertoire; we attend seminars that help us with personal discovery and spiritual growth.

Weekend workshops can reenergize us and give us new ideas and techniques to explore. Personal growth workshops can free us to have healthier relationships with ourselves and our clients. But these short courses can also give fresh meaning to the phrase "A little knowledge is a dangerous thing." Sometimes weekend workshops produce "instant experts." I've seen people with a weekend workshop or two under their belts doing cervical adjustments, giving advice on neurological problems, practicing pseudo-psychology, or claiming to understand the causes of cancer. These are dangerous presumptions of expertise.

We need to feel secure in the value of our training and our work. We need to realize that the ability to give a good massage or bodywork session is as good as gold and a good somatic practitioner enhances the quality of clients' lives every day. We don't need to embellish our skills or knowledge. If we do what we're trained to do competently and with compassion, it's more than enough.

We don't need to embellish our skills or knowledge. If we do what we're trained to do competently and with compassion, it's more than enough.

Some examples of what should stay outside the therapeutic circle are provided next.

Medical Advice

Pain science has advanced rapidly in recent years. There are more research studies on massage therapy than ever before, although assuredly, not everyone keeps currently with that knowledge—but they should. Training for massage therapists has become somewhat more standardized as more states have become regulated, although there is still a lot of variance in education from one school to another. Testing for a massage license is meant to insure that an entry-level massage therapist has basic knowledge required to safely practice massage. Because of these advances, we can be confused about our role in dealing with medical situations. True, sometimes somatic practitioners have resolved physical problems that have stumped physicians, but that does not mean that we are medical experts.

A group of bodyworkers were discussing a colleague's prospective client who had a rare disorder of the thoracic spine. Much advice was given about which vertebral muscles to work with, which to avoid, and how to help the client. Everyone's intentions were clearly good, but all these suggestions came from practitioners who had never seen the client and knew nothing of her history or the severity of her problem. Nor did any of them have the required training to work with a client with this rare disorder! It seems to be a phenomenon on social media that any time anyone says "I have such-and-such condition," or "My client has such-and-such condition," the advice—again, much of which is absurd and some of which is potentially harmful—starts rolling in—regardless of the fact that the people giving that advice know nothing more about the client, the medications they might be taking, the underlying pathology, the contraindications they may have, and so on. It seems that everyone thinks what they do is the best thing for it: "Get a Bowen session!" "She needs craniosacral!" "One session of (*insert modality*) would fix that!" Again, people have good intentions—and in many cases—very misguided good intentions.

Within the profession, there is concern about practitioners who treat medical issues without sufficient training or without consultation with the client's doctor or other involved practitioner. Such boundary violations can be as simple as giving advice that is traditionally in the medical realm; for instance, advising a client to give up an ankle brace or to cut back on medication. Or, these violations can be as dangerous as working with a client who has a serious medical condition, without permission and input from the appropriate medical practitioner. If medical doctors saw even a tenth of the advice given out by massage therapists on Facebook, none of them would ever make a referral to a massage therapist—particularly those who feel compelled to slam the medical profession and/or pharmaceuticals at every turn. Brent Jackson, program director of a massage therapy program that includes hospital-based massage, related the story of a therapist who was being interviewed for a job by hospital personnel. When asked about her motivations for doing this particular type of work, she responded with "I can't wait to get in the room and tell those patients what kind of poison the doctors are putting in their bodies!"

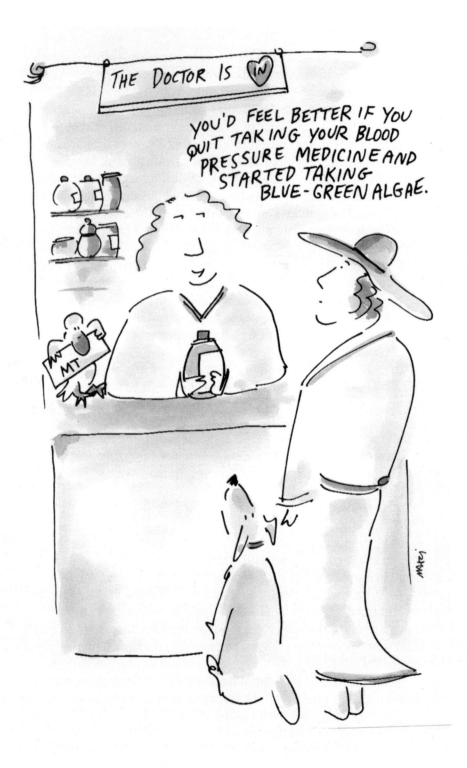

No, she did not get that job—hardly surprising! One therapist, in regard to the claims she was making about the essential oils she sells, when I mentioned the fact that the company she represents was reprimanded by the FDA for making false medical claims in their advertising, said "Of course the FDA will never approve of anything that actually helps people." Why would a doctor want to make a referral to someone like that? Very simple—they don't.

If we give an opinion, we need to identify it as a personal opinion unless it is within our scope of practice and training. Also, we need to take care how we state an opinion. "I've been using vitamin C for my own colds for years and its helped me," is safer to say than "You should take vitamin C."

Beyond a concern for staying out of legal hot water, we want to honor the dictum "First, do no harm." Although we can sometimes relieve a condition that wasn't helped by the usual medical regimen of drugs or surgery, that doesn't mean that we can hang out a shingle that reads, "The Doctor Is In." Most clients already give us more authority than is rightfully ours. It's up to us to stay honest and within the bounds of what we know and are authorized by the law to do.

Psychological Counseling

The hardest judgment calls to make about boundaries are those that concern psychological and emotional issues. When are we being friendly, and when are we making a mistake by acting like amateur psychotherapists? As practitioners, it's appropriate to be sensitive to our clients and supportive of them. It can be helpful to get to know them. Such information as whether a client exercises regularly, is happily partnered, or has a stressful job can give us a broader picture of the client and help us know how to work with them better. Except for obtaining information necessary for treatment, though, it's never appropriate to pry into a client's private life.

Many clients volunteer information about their lives and concerns, making it difficult for us to know how to respond. But we have to watch that we don't stumble into the role of psychotherapist or counselor by giving advice or counseling when we don't have the training. In general, anytime our response goes beyond good listening, we're probably heading down the wrong road. An exception would be if someone tells you they are being abused; then a comment such as "Are you aware of the Women's Shelter on 4th Street? They can help you get out of the situation you are in," and *stop there*. If someone confides in you, he or she is seriously depressed and doesn't know how to cope with it, then a comment such as "Dr. Collins has helped my friend deal with her depression. His office is in the Medical Building beside the hospital," is appropriate. It's always a good idea to know other professionals to refer to.

Counseling is more than just common sense. Without the appropriate education, we can't usually tell the difference between, for instance, a mentally disturbed person and someone who is reacting to a momentary or temporary crisis. We also don't usually have the training and fine-tuning it takes to keep our own biases and emotional reactions out of interactions with clients.

It can be easy to fall into the trap of naively giving advice about personal matters. Our motivation is good: we want to help our clients. After all, we have our accumulated personal experience, we've read books, and maybe we've been in therapy ourselves. We may have had emotional openings that were useful or even profound. We care about our clients; we see their unhappiness and want to share our experiences and philosophies with them.

Despite their good intentions, somatic practitioners who try to act like counselors are often clumsy—doing things that a good (trained) psychotherapist would not do, such as giving advice, confronting clients bluntly, or making hasty interpretations without really knowing a client. Even if we have training in these areas, we must look at the reason the client has come to us. If he or she comes to us for a painful lower back, it's not our business to tell him or her that he or she may be angry with his or her boss. However, in our role as educators, we could say, for instance, "Muscle tension is often related to our anxiety about a problem. Perhaps, you've been under stress at work or at home."

On the other hand, sometimes we interpret our unspoken contract too strictly. For instance, some practitioners are uncomfortable when clients want to talk about their personal lives; they believe it isn't their job to listen to even the minor issues of a client's daily life. They want to interpret the contract very narrowly and say, "I only work with muscles." But isn't it part of our professional role to provide an atmosphere within which clients can relax those tight muscles? Some clients unwind by talking. This may be especially true of those who live alone, and maybe lacking in social interaction. Although it's not our job to give advice or counseling, we can provide a sympathetic ear.

Spiritual Advice

➤ *A client who was going through a rough time in her life complained to her new massage therapist about how difficult things were for her. The next time she saw the massage therapist, she was startled and a little put off when the therapist handed her a religious pamphlet of inspirational stories.*

Regardless of how meaningful a spiritual path or religious group has been to us, it's not appropriate to set ourselves up as spiritual advisors. That's not part of our job description or our scope of practice. If a client is on a much different path than you are, even having a conversation about it in the treatment room can be divisive and make for bad feelings on the part of either or both parties. What if the client is a fundamentalist Christian, and you are an atheist, or vice versa? That conversation is probably not going to work out well. Having a religious debate in the massage space is not going to be a relaxing experience for the client—or the therapist. One therapist related the story that a new client asked her right after the massage began if she was "saved." When the therapist answered that she was a nonbeliever, the client started crying and praying aloud that the therapist would accept Jesus. The therapist continued on with the session, which in reality, was uncomfortable for both of them.

Some people deliberately seek health-care providers or service providers of the same faith, or even the specific church they go to, while to do so may never cross the mind of others. People have the right to seek services from anyone they choose, but it would be discrimination on the part of a therapist to limit his or her clients only to Christians or any other group. You can hardly hang out a sign that says "Pagans Only" on the front of your business. Nor should you try to talk to clients into adopting your own spiritual or religious belief system (or lack of one)—ever.

In the same vein, some therapists may not realize that even the atmosphere in their office may be off-putting to some clients. If you walked into a business you had never patronized before, and all the artwork was religious in nature, and the table in the waiting room was covered in religious pamphlets and a stack of pocket-sized Bibles with a sign encouraging you to take one, would you feel comfortable? What if there was a huge statue of the Buddha in the waiting room, a pentagram, or representations of symbols you don't know the meaning of painted on the walls? Would you feel comfortable, or would you feel that you might have chosen the wrong place to spend your money? Put yourself in the client's place. You're not going to a doctor to get spiritual advice, and the public is not coming to you to get spiritual advice.

Mixing Other Businesses with Our Practice

> *A massage therapist who had an outside part-time office job gave her boss a massage, not knowing that he was having marital problems with his wife, who also worked in the office. As clients sometimes do, during the massage, he began to confide in her about his unhappiness with his wife. The massage therapist felt awkward about hearing these confidences and didn't know if the boss was subtly expressing interest in her. After that encounter, she became uneasy in a work situation that had previously been comfortable.*

Problems can arise from mixing business transactions—either taking on business associates as clients or trying to involve our clients in other kinds of business transactions. The former can lead, as it did in the above example, to a confusion of roles, and the latter can have results that are harmful and even unethical. We might sell a supplement to a client who then has an allergic reaction to it, or sell a weight-loss product to a client who doesn't lose any weight (never mind that they might not have seen the tiny print that tells them they have to exercise and stick to 1,000 calories a day, too). Or, more likely, we may lose a client because he or she doesn't like being pressured to buy our magnets, supplements, or whatever other product we might be selling. Unfortunately, some employers ask (or even require) their massage therapists to aggressively sell products to clients—going so far as to give them scripts to repeat to the client and training in how to sell. Be sure you know company policies on this issue before you sign a contract.

The most serious consideration is that it's unethical to use our relationships with clients to benefit ourselves in ways other than our standard fees. Clients make themselves vulnerable to us and appreciate us because of the unselfish role that we take on as their practitioner. We take advantage of that vulnerability when we try to use our influence to persuade clients to buy certain products or engage in business with us in other ways.

Boundaries Aren't Barriers

Boundaries aren't barriers between practitioner and client. Every relationship in our lives has boundaries. These limits tell us what to expect and what's appropriate in a particular situation. Boundaries are a natural part of everyone's world. The old adage, "Good fences make for good neighbors," can be paraphrased here: *good boundaries make for good therapeutic relationships*.

Boundaries help keep us within the limits of our training. They keep our egos in check and our insecurities out of our sessions, and they keep us honest. By maintaining good boundaries, we can show the best of ourselves. Good boundaries are at the heart of being a skillful and compassionate practitioner. They are what makes us professional in the eyes of the world and bring respectability and credibility to our work.

Questions for Reflection

1. Make a case for why keeping good boundaries helps clients feel safe and comfortable with us and why it matters that clients feel safe. If you don't believe that clients need to feel safe or that good boundaries help, defend that position.

2. A client tells you that she has been having an affair for the past several years with a married man who has repeatedly promised to leave his wife but has never done so. She says she doesn't know what to do and seems confused and upset. As her massage therapist, how can you respond without crossing boundaries?

3. Think back to your first professional massage. (If you haven't had a professional massage, stop right now and go get one.) Were you nervous? Did you know what to expect? Is there anything the practitioner could have told

you either on the phone or when you first arrived that could have made you more comfortable or that would have helped you know what to expect?

4. Has a professional of any kind ever given you advice that was outside his or her level of expertise and also unasked for? How did you feel about that? Did you address it with him or her in any way? Did you return for another visit?

5. A client who has never had a massage before has low back pain. You failed to explain to her that the session would involve working on the gluts. She seemed to be enjoying the massage until you touched her gluteals, at which point in time you felt her flinch and stiffen up on the table. What will you say to make up for your previous lack of clear communication? What if she is uncomfortable with you working there, even after you have explained how the gluteals are involved?

---

thePoint To learn more about the concepts discussed in this chapter, visit http://thePoint .lww.com/Allen-McIntosh4e

CHAPTER 3

Framework: Nuts and Bolts of Boundaries

Framework:
The logistics by which we define ourselves as professionals and create a safe atmosphere for our clients. Framework includes the ways that we present ourselves in advertising, the preparation of the physical setting, our policies on fees and time, and such ground rules as keeping the focus on the client.

Framework details are the nuts and bolts of good boundaries.

Framework issues can seem dry and dull. Who wants to talk about the joy of starting sessions on time and the delights of clean sheets? But it is in those details that we define our practices as professional. As discussed in previous chapters, our clients are vulnerable; they need good boundaries to trust us. Framework details are the nuts and bolts of good boundaries.

This list could go on for an entire chapter, but you get the picture. Giving a good massage is just *one* facet of the total therapeutic relationship. The nuts and bolts can make it or break it.

Our clients know little about the technical part of our work. Our offices are foreign territory to them. The only way they can judge our competence and caring is by our professional behavior and whether they feel safe with us. The ability to create an atmosphere within which clients can make use of our work is crucial. We may rush to learn the latest techniques and pride ourselves on our sensitivity, but our effectiveness may depend on whether or not the nuts and bolts are taken care of.

If you work at a spa or in a doctor's office, you may have limited control over some aspects of framework discussed later, such as the decor of the treatment room or how clients are scheduled. However, other guidelines, such as not discussing clients' treatment with them outside of your work environment, are relevant no matter where you practice.

The Need for Framework: Holding the Space

Some practitioners call it "holding the space." Others call it "creating a container." They recognize that clients need to have a special environment that is focused solely on their well-being. Attending to framework is more than simply buying

CONSIDER THIS

Many somatic practitioners' careers have suffered because of carelessness about the finer points that make clients comfortable. Clients care about those issues more than we may be aware. The quality of care that someone receives from us means more than just giving a good massage.

Many times, what makes a client leave a therapist has nothing to do with whether or not they give a good massage; sometimes, it's the framework—*the nuts and bolts*—of the business. Some of the reasons clients give for leaving one therapist and seeking another—many times prefaced with a statement like "She gave a good massage, but. . . _____."

- The bathroom at her office was just plain dirty.
- Her treatment room was so cluttered it looked like a garage sale.
- She never really seemed to be listening to me when I was telling her what was wrong.
- She had an earpiece and answered the phone during my massage.
- She would just sit there holding her hands on me. I don't know what she was doing.
- She's always running late. My massage never starts on time.
- She only had one hand on me and was texting someone.
- The music she played was creepy.
- She is always calling me to reschedule my appointment because "something personal has come up."
- The sheets smelled funny.
- I was uncomfortable getting a massage in a room that only had one candle burning and no other light.
- She talked my ear off about her children and her personal problems.
- She dropped several hints that I should leave a tip.
- She talked about other clients to me, so I figured she'd talk to them about me.
- Her clothes smelled like cigarettes.
- Her office smelled like a perfume factory and I never have liked the smell of lavender.
- I was uncomfortable with the bolster under my knees and she said I had to have it.
- She just wasn't very friendly.
- She's always trying to sell me something I don't want.
- She's always dressed sloppy and barefooted.
- She keeps asking me to come to her church.
- Her cat was in the office and there was cat hair around and a litter box in the front office.

massage oil and soothing music; we need to take care of all the details that make us professional. Careless framework can interfere with the therapeutic process. A colleague reports:

➤ *I used to be a massage therapist in a holistic center in which no one had an assigned office. Instead, we used whatever room was available at the time. Sometimes my client and I had to wait 10 or 15 minutes until a room was free. We rarely worked in the same room two times in a row. The other practitioners and I often talked about how uptight our clients seemed to be. Now I see that their difficulty letting go was probably a response to our erratic setup. How could they relax in such an unstable environment?*

Boundary Lessons

I was working in a group practice (we were all renting space together) with several other massage therapists, one of whom was going to be out of work for several weeks due to a minor surgery. She told several of her regular clients that she recommended they see me while she was recovering. At the end of the session with the first one, she said "I don't want to hurt her feelings, but I'd rather see you again. She gives a great massage but she talks the whole time, and I just want to rest and relax." A couple of the other people she had referred to me rebooked with me, saying virtually the same thing. I didn't know what to say to the other therapist, who was expecting those clients to be rebooked with her when she returned. We weren't really close friends, but we were always cordial at the office and frequently ate in the break room together. I didn't want to hurt her feelings, either, but I felt she was going to be offended if I said anything to her, not to mention being worried about violating confidentiality by repeating what the clients had said. It came to a head the first day she dropped into the office during her recovery and saw the appointment book. She said "I'm coming back to work on the 15th, my clients can see me." When I told her they had requested to stay with me, she got mad, accused me of stealing her clients, and stomped out of the office. She called me later, still mad, and I suggested that *she* call the clients and let them know she was back at work, and *they* told her they had requested to see me again. She stuck around for a few weeks and ignored me at work, and the other therapists there took it on themselves to talk to her about her attitude and tell her she was making the atmosphere of whole office miserable. They pointed out to her that clients have the right to see anyone they choose and that we do not have ownership of clients. She refused to back down on her stance that I had stolen her clients, and shortly after that, ended up leaving the office and working by herself.

REAL EXPERIENCE

A popular massage therapist worked for years out of a room in her home that was less than neat—in fact, it was a cluttered mess. Despite that, she was successful because she was a good listener and a sensitive bodyworker, plus she was professional in every other way. Recently, she complained that her work seemed to take more and more energy over the years. I suggested that she try simply tidying up the room. I thought that she wouldn't have to work as hard to create a professional atmosphere if the room said it for her. It was a small change, but she reported that cleaning up the room made a difference. She looks forward to her work more in this neater, more professional office and reports that new clients seem to settle in and relax faster.

When the framework isn't stable, sometimes clients are uncomfortable without knowing why. They just feel out of kilter. They may be more demanding or more tense than they would be if they felt safe and attended to. Practitioners also are affected by unreliable framework. Not only are we more likely to be dealing with cranky clients, but also we can be drained by the lack of stability in our work lives.

There *are* good practitioners who are careless with framework, yet seem to have healthy practices. Clients sometimes forgive other omissions if the practitioner has a terrific personality or great technical skills. Yet, even in those cases, clients notice and respond positively if those practitioners start attending to framework issues. Also, the practitioners find they have fewer "difficult" clients and more energy at the end of the day.

Some practitioners have great personalities or amazing skills. For the rest of us, the majority, who are charismatically impaired and less-than-dazzling technicians, attention to framework balances our shortcomings. Consistency, care for the client, and the ability to set limits well can go a long way toward a solid, satisfying practice. And we will last longer in this profession.

Framework Basics: Setting the Stage

Our work with clients begins long before they walk through the door. It starts with the first phone call, the first time they meet us, or even the first time they see our business card. We need to take care of how we present ourselves from the very beginning. With every detail, we need to consider the basics of the professional therapeutic relationship. For instance, any advertising—whether it's putting up a business card at the health food store, running an ad in the newspaper, or creating a website—should involve clear and honest information about who we are and what we do. Ads are the beginning of educating clients about what to expect from us.

Business Cards

Business cards usually won't make or break a practice. Some practitioners with successful practices have unimpressive-looking cards. However, your card is one more piece of information about you; you want it to give clients a favorable impression and perhaps a sense of your personal style.

CONSIDER THIS

What does the name of your business (and subsequently, your advertising) convey about you? Does it convey the impression you really want to give people? If you specialize in orthopedic massage and wish to have a more medically-oriented massage practice, then "Hands of Light" is not going to get that message across—but "Meyer Orthopedic Massage Therapy" leaves no doubt about what it is you do. Choosing a name because it has sentimental significance to you is okay, but again, you need to be certain that it conveys the message. Perhaps you grew up in Australia, and "kookaburra," which is an Australian bird, was a nickname given to you when you were a lad, so you decide to name your business "Kookaburra Kare." People are not going to have any idea what that is unless you add the words "Massage Therapy" to that. Maybe you're fond of collecting unicorns. "Unicorn Massage Therapy" conveys that it's a massage business, but on the other hand, it doesn't sound like a medical massage practice—which is fine, if you're not attempting to convey the image of a medical massage practitioner.

If you name your massage practice "The Zen Center," you need to keep in mind that (a) some people may not know what Zen means (it refers to a Buddhist practice of meditation), and (b) people who are familiar with the term may assume that it's a meditation center. While massage can induce a meditative state, if you want to be sure people know you're running a massage practice, then "The Zen Massage Center" would be a better choice.

You might also think twice about using cutesy names, such as "We Knead U." The tone is friendly and humorous but could be seen as making a joke of your work. While "Rub a Dub" is lighthearted, without the words "Massage Therapy" added to that, people may take that to mean you're washing cars for a living. If you're just starting out in business, give careful consideration to the message you really want to send to potential clients. Making a mistake in your choice of business name can be expensive, both in costing you your business because people don't really understand from the name of the business what services you are offering, and in having to pay to reprint all your business and advertising materials once reality has set in that it wasn't a good choice.

Business cards should be simple and eye catching. Avoid making a long list of the techniques and modalities you offer, especially if they are techniques that are unfamiliar to most of the public. Some cards look like a smorgasbord: "Mary Smith—Hypnotherapy, Past Life Regression, Acupressure, Sports Massage, Doula Services, Reflexology, and Palm Reading." That hodgepodge of services can be bewildering to the public, and prospective clients could also be skeptical that, unless Mary Smith is 103 years old, she can't be really good at all of those things.

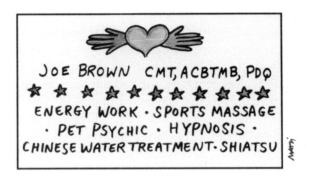

Beware of using only your first name on a business card. It may look as though you have a reason to hide your identity, and it's also the way that sex workers frequently advertise on Craig's List or in the newspaper. Not a good idea. Having a business card shows people that you're serious about your work; people expect professionals to have business cards. Also, the process of designing a card often helps you clarify what tone you want to set for your business and what you want people to know about you.

Advertising and Reaching the Public

If you wish to advertise, there are some basic guidelines to follow. It may sound obvious, but first decide what population you want to reach and then figure out how to contact them. It's a good idea to talk with colleagues and more experienced practitioners in your area to see what has worked for them. As with business cards, advertising needs to be simple and attractive. Massage is such a personal service that you may not receive many calls from impersonal advertising alone, but it does help prospective clients to begin to associate your name with your business.

Speaking to groups about massage is one good way to advertise. Civic groups such as the Rotary Club or Lions Club are always looking for interesting speakers, and they usually only want you to speak for a short time, not give a dissertation. Once people have met you (assuming you appear friendly and professional), they are more likely to feel comfortable making an appointment. Such presentations can include a short talk on the benefits of massage or your particular kind of massage, followed by a brief demonstration. The demonstration can be, for instance, a foot massage on a clothed volunteer. It helps if people can see the care and concern with which you approach your clients. Your talk can include enough technical detail or anatomical references to show people that you know what you are doing; however, keep in mind that most people just want to know if you can help them feel better.

Websites

For those in private practice, having a website has become practically a necessity for connecting with prospective clients. Unlike business cards and ads, websites give you room to explain your kind of bodywork, credentials, fees and office policies, and answers to typical concerns. You can put your website's address on your business card and give prospective clients the opportunity to find out more about you. A website doesn't need to be elaborate and large—just attractive, professional, and informative. It's another way to convey your own style and values. As with any advertising, it's a good idea to get feedback from colleagues and mentors before making it official.

It's time to bring up the subject of social media again. Many people now have Facebook pages, Twitter accounts, or other social media pages that they use for their business. Some people may talk about their business on their personal Facebook page, or mention something about their personal life on their business page. There's a lot of overlap.

If you are identifying yourself as a massage therapist on your Facebook page, ask yourself how you would be perceived if a client saw your page. Are you posting pictures of yourself at the beach, showing off the rear view of you in your thong, or looking sloppy drunk at a concert? That's not a good idea, and you shouldn't be surprised if you get phone calls wanting to know if you provide that *other* kind of massage.

Yes, Facebook does have privacy settings. However, in this day and age, we should probably all assume that everything we do in public (and sometimes in private) is on the Internet for the world to see. Remember, many of the pictures and videos on the Internet are unauthorized, taken by someone with a phone that you didn't even know was watching you, much less consider that they'd post your picture or video on *their* Facebook page.

Being friends with your clients on social media is also a potentially troublesome. Do you really want your clients to see everything you post, from your political views to pictures of your high school prom? Or irreverent, rude, or profane comments from your friends? Keep in mind that if you allow your clients on your personal page, and your friend, who has his own privacy settings so that anyone can see *his* posts—or may even be a friend of your client—puts up that picture of your wild night at the bachelor party on his page and tags you in it, well, there you are.

Phone and Voice Mail Guidelines

If clients call you directly to set up appointments, what they hear when they first call your business phone number is an important part of setting the stage. Very few independent practitioners have an office with a receptionist. Most have various ways—such as voice mail and answering machines—for people to contact them and leave messages. No matter what your preference, you want to be easily accessible, sound professional, and provide privacy for your clients and prospective clients. This is often the first contact the public has with you, and you don't want it to be the last.

I once called a former student of mine when I was passing through her town, and got her office voice mail. Very loud reggae music was playing in the background, and she was giggling throughout the message. It really came across as if she was drunk—and I left her a message to that effect. It's also unprofessional—and nobody thinks it's cute except you—to have your 4-year-old record your message. Would you have confidence in a doctor's professionalism if a 4-year-old answered the office phone? No, you wouldn't. Remember, you only get one chance to make a first impression.

Be certain that your greeting message is also professional when you're leaving an out-of-the-office message. Just yesterday, I called a therapist and got the message "I'm on vacation. Leave me a message." Not so much as her name or the business name, no hint of when she would return or would be returning calls. A first-time caller, or even a regular client who is in a pain crisis, will probably call someone else if they have no clue when you might be getting back to them.

Right from the start, you can (and should) demonstrate the elements of a professional relationship. For instance, to be client centered in your first contact, put yourself in the client's position. What kind of message would you want to hear if you were calling a stranger to ask him or her to work with you in a highly personal way?

For clients' confidentiality, you need to have a way that they can leave a message that only you can access.

Other boundaries come into play here. For clients' confidentiality, you need to have a way that they can leave a message that only you can access.

If your phone line is shared with colleagues, family members, or others, it is easy to have a separate box to your answering system and a message of "Press 1 to leave a message for Susan Jones or press 2 to leave a message for Donna Barker." Alternately, a voice mail service or cell phone exclusively for your business is a good choice. These options also avoid the boundary problem of giving clients an unnecessary glimpse into your private life. Even if you live in a small town and everyone knows a good deal about your personal life, prospective clients will be comforted to know that you keep your business separate and guard your clients' privacy.

It's unprofessional and a violation of confidentiality to allow client's messages to be heard by your family members or anyone other than staff members who are trained to keep confidentiality. Even the fact that someone is your client should be guarded. A colleague reports:

> ➤ *I once worked with a small group of therapists and bodyworkers in a situation where everyone shared a phone line and each of us could hear the others' messages as they looked for their own. More than once, I heard parts of private messages that I'm sure the person wouldn't have wanted me to hear. Just the sound of a client's voice when that person is feeling needy is too personal for your colleague, partner, or family member to hear.*

Your phone greetings should be warm but businesslike and to the point: "You've reached Michael Wallace, Massage Therapist. Please leave your name and number and a brief message, and I'll return your call." And does anyone really enjoy having to listen to a musical prelude when they reach someone's answering machine? Some people may think your Mozart on Muzak is lovely, while the rock and roll fan may find it irritating. Prospective clients usually appreciate a short, relevant, friendly message.

If you take and return business calls from your home, make sure the television isn't blaring in the background, your dog isn't barking, and your children aren't yelling for your attention. For incoming calls, use a screening device such as a caller ID so you can choose when to answer. Allowing friends and family members to answer your business calls can lead to problems. For instance, a boyfriend answering the phone may send out more information about your life than the client needs. And a small child answering the phone might be endearing but also annoying. Even 1 minute of repeating "Is your mommy home?" may give new clients second thoughts about making an appointment with a new practitioner. They may wonder if the practitioner's family life will interfere with her professional life in other ways.

The First Conversation

The therapeutic relationship starts with the first conversation.

The therapeutic relationship starts with the first conversation. If you have a private practice, the first conversation will usually be on the phone. In a spa or a doctor's office, it will generally be in person.

Private Practice: The Initial Phone Conversation

When a prospective client calls to ask about your work, be informative and reassuring, but don't sound as if you're reading from a set speech. Know ahead of time how you want to answer the usual questions: your fees, your hours, and the particular benefits of your modality. (Chapter 8 gives tips about how to deal with clients looking for sexual services as well as how to advertise to avoid such misunderstandings.) Most massage schools now have student clinics, where students may take turns in performing massage and working the desk; some also have internship opportunities where further experience in customer service skills are taught. If that was not the case at your school, it's a good idea to ask more experienced colleagues in their area for advice about this first phone call. Also, you don't want to stumble around when prospective clients ask you the benefits of your work. Rehearse with a friend. Avoid making false claims, such as the tired myth about massage releasing toxins from the body, or promising people that a massage is the cure for whatever ails them. While we like to think that massage is good for everything, it's simply not true.

Much can be learned about clients in the initial phone call. Do they, for instance, want to share a great deal of personal information or ask for advice? You can start setting boundaries in that first call by letting them know that some issues are best dealt with during office visits. Be careful about letting people take up an unusual amount of time on the phone; it sets a bad precedent. Even with these earliest contacts, it's important to be aware of setting limits to protect yourself.

If a client asks for an appointment tomorrow at 3 p.m. and you don't have that opening, you don't need to apologize and ramble on, as if to a friend, about why you can't see them then. Clients simply want to know what appointment you *do* have open.

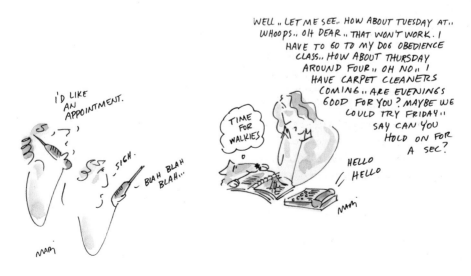

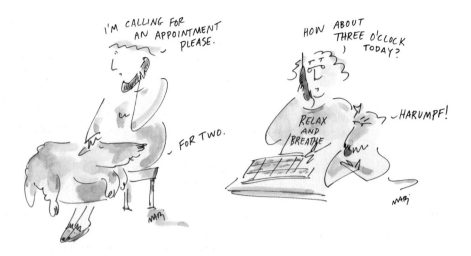

The first phone call is a great opportunity to educate the client. You can set the stage for the session. It's a good idea to ask the caller if he or she has had massage before; if not, explain what will happen in the session very thoroughly so that there's no mystery. Let the client know that you will take a health history, and explain to him or her that it is in order to be sure that he or she has no contraindications for massage (and in regulated states, it's required by law). Let him or her know that you will then leave the room so that he or she can get undressed, that the person will lie under a sheet and be draped at all times, and so forth. Let the client know from the beginning that if he or she is uncomfortable in any way, at any time, that you want him or her to speak up right away. Aside from honoring clients' right to informed consent, letting new clients know what to expect can help them be more at ease when they arrive for their first session.

Any client who is put off or indignant about having to give health history must be educated to the reasons you are asking. The general public is not aware that there are contraindications and cautions for massage, which is why we have to be, and why we're obligated to let them know. In regulated states, it's also the law.

Working for an Employer: The First In-Person Encounter

If you work for a spa, physician, or chiropractor—basically any setting in which the client has been assigned to you without first meeting you—you may have only a brief time in which to orient clients to the setting and put them at ease, perhaps only the moments between meeting a client in the reception area and walking him or her to the treatment room. Still, that's time enough for you to establish the beginnings of trust. It may be inadequate, however, to conduct a proper intake interview; so if you see anything of concern on their intake form, you may need to question them a little more once they're in the treatment room.

Remember that most clients may be unsure about what to expect; they may not have been to your spa or place of employment before and they may never have had a massage. As much as possible, spell things out for them: "I'm glad to be working with you today. We'll go back to the treatment room and I'll tell you more about what to expect." One massage therapist at a spa noticed that clients seemed wary when she closed the door to talk with them. When she started explaining to new clients, "I'm closing the door to keep the noise out while we talk," that settled them down.

Simple and clear explanations are helpful: "This is the private room where I'll work with you. In a minute, I'll leave while you undress and get under the sheet, and we'll be starting with you face up, please" (some clients may not be familiar with the term *supine*). "But first, I want to know if you have any particular place that is tense or hurting you, like your shoulders or back?"

Remember that this can be a foreign setting for many people and the issue of nudity can make them anxious. Explain to them that they will be covered with a sheet during the massage, except for where you are working, and that they can fully undress or leave on underwear for their comfort. Most people want to do what's appropriate. They just need to know exactly what you expect.

Framework Basics: The Setting

A therapy room that feels safe, clean, and uncluttered will seem inviting to clients, will benefit your practice, and be a joy for you to work in.

Private Practice: Home or Office?

Where to locate a private practice is a personal choice that depends on several factors, including cost and convenience. If you can afford it, working out of an office rather than a home is generally more professional, and will feel safer both to you and to your clients. A client reports:

➤ *When I first started getting bodywork, I made an appointment with a male practitioner I didn't know. Even though he'd been well recommended, I was a little uncomfortable because he worked out of his house, which turned out to be at the end of a long driveway off the highway. When I went for that first appointment, I actually gave a friend the practitioner's address and said, "If I don't call you in 2 hours, call the police." The session went fine, but I want bodyworkers to know that their business can be affected if they work out of their homes.*

If you choose to work out of your home, use a room that's set aside just for your professional work. The message to clients is that this is a space solely for clients.

There's also an advantage to being able to shut the office door at the end of your business day and focus on your private life without reminders of work concerns.

When working out of your home, the best arrangement is to have a separate entrance for clients or a way for them to access your office without getting a view of your private living space. Having a separate bathroom for clients is also ideal. If you don't have a separate entrance and separate bathroom to your massage space, you have to be very mindful of clients walking through your home. If you have children, be sure there are no toys left around that a client could trip over, no Legos in the floor for them to step on as they walk to the bathroom, and no dirty diapers smelling up the bathroom trash can. If you're using your home for an office, you have to keep it as clean and sanitary as you would if you were practicing in a professional setting.

Whether your office is in your home or in another location, you want it to feel warm and inviting to your clients but still professional and not overwhelmingly personal. If you work out of your home, you don't want your office space to look like a bedroom with a massage table in it—eliminate bedroom-type furniture and large numbers of personal pictures and items. There's no harm in having a family picture in the room—in fact, it can be reassuring to clients to see that a practitioner is coupled or has children. Also, a picture of the practitioner's partner or spouse may discourage a client from making romantic overtures.

Practitioners need to avoid making their offices into displays of their personal beliefs—political, spiritual, or otherwise. Clients may feel excluded if they don't share your beliefs, or they may have judgments about your beliefs that will affect how they feel about you.

Preparing the Room

Wherever you work, clients love coming into a room that's all set up for them—neat, clean sheets on the table and everything ready to go. Ready rooms are an immediate sign of your professionalism and caring. Extra touches like a table warmer, fleece pad, and a robe for the client to slip on should they feel the need to go to the bathroom, are appreciated.

Clients won't feel comfortable in unclean rooms or surroundings. Make sure the treatment room and the bathroom clients will use are clean. With so many new viruses and bacteria popping up these days, people are concerned about catching something. Find a balance between a room that smells antiseptic and one that feels as though germs may be lurking in every corner. (Also, remember to wash your hands before and after you work with a client. Although that sounds obvious, if doctors forget to do it—and studies show that they do—manual therapists probably do, too.) The need for order and cleanliness in the environment can go deeper for some clients. After all, some people grow up with ideas about their bodies being "dirty" and may feel a heightened sensitivity when they come for bodywork. Clean, orderly surroundings help clients relax.

There's a saying, "Heaven is in the details." Professionalism calls for an angelic attention to the finer aspects of how you present yourself and your work and how you welcome clients into your practice.

Draping

Appropriate draping of clients is required for privacy and comfort. If a client asks not to be draped, advise the client that it's part of your professional standards that every client be draped—and in all regulated states, it's the law. There's no really good reason to allow a client not to be draped. The manual therapy profession is still striving to separate its public image from that of sex workers, and appropriate draping is an easy way you can define that difference. Draping is meant to ensure the modesty, safety, and comfort of the client—and is a safeguard for the massage therapist as well. You might not be able to keep a professional demeanor if someone's private parts are staring you in the face for the whole session.

Many state boards have written into their rules a statement such as "the drape may be temporarily removed in order to apply treatment." Be as diligent in honoring the client's modesty as possible. For example, if you're working the client's gluteal muscles, only expose one side at a time—don't pull the whole drape down to leave them uncovered.

Basic Session Framework

Erratic framework affects both client and practitioner. Clients may feel nervous or fussy in a confused framework, and practitioners may respond by being harried or drained by the end of the day. For instance, imagine being careless with just one aspect of framework, such as starting and ending on time. How would you feel if you ran late all day? Imagine how it would feel to be the client of someone who was never on time. The following framework guidelines provide a solid structure for your work. (These guidelines were adapted from Narboe N. *Working with What You Can't Get Your Hands On*. Portland, OR: Narboe; 1985.) It's still timely advice. If these guidelines sound too much like rules, try thinking of them as small acts of kindness toward vulnerable clients. They are also small acts of self-discipline that will make your work life run more smoothly. If you aren't already using these guidelines, you may want to try them out and see if you notice a positive difference. (Practitioners who have been scattered about framework in the past will need to be consistently careful for some time before noticing a difference.) If you work for someone else, you may not have control over the implementation of some of these guidelines. Therefore, you may want to seek clarification about a prospective employer's policies, particularly on such issues as informed consent and confidentiality.

- Clients know what to expect and what is expected of them.
- Sessions start and end on time.

- Sessions occur at the same time and place at regular intervals.
- Nothing interrupts a session.
- Practitioners avoid casual discussion of treatment or sessions with clients outside office boundaries.
- Practitioners carefully safeguard clients' rights to privacy and confidentiality.
- Clients are unaware of each other.
- Practitioners don't ask clients to attend to their needs.

Clients Know What to Expect and What is Expected of Them

Before you begin the hands-on work, you need to receive the informed consent of the client. If you are in private practice, you can ask the client to sign a consent form that explains your credentials, the nature of the treatment, and the possible benefits and side effects. All massage therapists would be wise to advise the client in written or verbal form about any consequences of the treatment such as muscle soreness or light-headedness. Assure clients that they have the right to refuse any procedure at any time. Clients should also be advised during the session when you want to introduce any treatment procedure not previously agreed to and also when you are going to be working near the breasts, anus, or genitals.

The agreement the client signs should also give details about fees and cancellation policies and any other financial policies, such as procedures for returned checks. If you work for someone else, your employer is responsible for financial agreements. It's wise to have the client sign a form stating that they have been informed of, and agree to abide by, your policies. You may want to put the policies and signature line on the back of your intake forms.

Procedures regarding confidentiality should be part of the initial intake of those in private practice and are discussed under "Practitioners Carefully Safeguard Clients' Rights to Privacy and Confidentiality," later in this chapter.

Sessions Start and End on Time

Time boundaries help make a safe container—they define the professional situation as different from a social one and put limits on the nature of the relationship. Obviously, if you're in private practice, you'll have more control over the time variables; however, those who work for others can do their best to provide good time boundaries within the structure provided by their employer.

Starting on time is respectful of both your time and the client's. For instance, if a client shows up early for an appointment, you still want to start the session at the appointed time, unless you were genuinely just sitting there killing time until they arrive and would relish finishing earlier. Don't let a client cut into the time you've set aside to rest or return messages. If a client with a 3 p.m. appointment arrives at 2:45 p.m., and you are taking a needed break or attending to other business, you can greet her with a smile and say, "I see you're early. Please have a seat in the waiting area, and I'll be ready for you at 3 p.m." Or you might say "You're welcome to rest on the table for a few minutes, since you arrived early. I'll be with you at 3 p.m."

Ending on time is just as important. Clients like to know what to expect and schedule other parts of their lives based on those expectations. Unpredictable practitioners can make clients uneasy. If you go long one session because the client is in pain, she may think you'll go short next time if she's not and may begin to come up with a new pain at the end of each session, unless you communicate that clearly during the session. Don't just assume it's okay to keep on working; the client may have a pressing appointment after the session. There's also the question of compensation. You may say "I know you only scheduled an hour, but if you have the time to stretch that to 90 minutes today, I think that would be beneficial to you. It will cost $30 more for the extra time," or something similar.

Being consistent about time has many advantages for practitioners. If you're usually consistent but find yourself always wanting to go over or under the usual amount of time with a certain client, this can be a sign that you need to look at why you are treating that client differently. It also makes it easier to monitor yourself in other ways. If you want to take extra time with *every* client, you may be trying too hard, and if you want to cut the session short with every client, you may be approaching burnout. There are therapists who only offer 90-minute sessions; Nina McIntosh herself was a Rolfer, and those sessions usually take an hour and a half to two hours. Therapists who work in medical settings may routinely do 15 to 30 minutes "spot work." Whatever the schedule and the contracted agreement is, stick to it, unless any changes have been thoroughly discussed with the client.

Even if clients are still experiencing intense emotion or pain, ending close to the agreed-on time can provide comforting structure. Lengthening sessions a great deal because there is still pain or emotion could tell clients that you think you are responsible for their pain rather than that your job is to do your best within a certain time limit. It may also show that you don't trust that the work you've already done will have results or that your clients have other resources as well.

If you have any clients who have a pattern of requesting additional work at the end of a session, it might be a good idea to inform them how much time is left, perhaps about 10 minutes before the end of the session, and ask if they have any areas that need special attention during the remaining time. You may also say "I have another appointment scheduled, so I can't go over today; why don't we just book you for 90 minutes in the future? It will be an extra $30." That way, you have let them know you intend to stick with the schedule—and that if they want more time, they need to pay for it.

The meaning of "ending on time" varies from practitioner to practitioner. Many somatic practitioners don't schedule precisely on the hour or half hour; they allow for a little extra work time on the table, gathering-up time for slow-moving clients, or breathing room for themselves. The amount of time varies from practitioner to practitioner, but 15 extra minutes is usually enough leeway. Many franchise and spa employees are obligated to do 50-minute massage these days, and there is inadequate time to regroup before the next client. Being consistent about time doesn't mean that you need to be rigid; sometimes a client is in an unusual crisis. A massage therapist told of taking an extra 30 minutes with a client whose mother had just died. (The therapist wasn't disrupting other clients' schedules by doing so.) A bodyworker said she scheduled extra time with a client who had come a long distance to work with her. Also, if *you* are late to a session, you want to make up that time to the client, either that day or at a later time.

It's also a good idea, even if your practice isn't full, to schedule and end sessions on time as if you were solidly booked. It's good discipline, and it shows clients that you value your time. Your practice will run much more smoothly, and your clients will be more secure.

Sessions Occur at the Same Time and Place at Regular Intervals

Although you're not in control of whether your clients come back regularly, be aware of the importance of consistency and try to keep regular clients in the same time slot. If you have to bounce a client out of a regular time or if you're relocating your practice to a different office, you want to be aware of keeping the other parts of the framework on an even keel. Moves and changes can upset clients without their fully realizing it. While this won't apply to sporadic clients and tourists passing through, it makes regular clients feel special when you try to be consistent with their schedule; it also helps them remain in better ease between sessions, and helps you in planning your income and your own work schedule.

If you work for a spa or a doctor's office, you might try to educate your employer about the importance of consistency for clients (delicately; some employers may have the attitude that you're a disruptive employee who is trying to tell them how to run the business). If you felt comfortable doing so, you could let your boss or the scheduler know that you'd like to work with regular clients in the same therapy room each time, for instance.

When you do have to see clients at a time other than their usual appointment time, or when you move to a new office or work out of a different treatment room, you may notice that some clients behave differently—they may be pickier, more off-balance, more insecure in some way. You may have to make an extra effort to help them feel comfortable. You could make a comment to show them that you understand how unsettling such an adjustment can be. For instance, if they're acting rattled, you could say, "It must feel strange to come in at a different time (or be in a new office)."

Nothing Interrupts a Session

All of these guidelines are based on the central idea that being professional means that the focus is on the client. Clients are paying for your time and attention. You don't want your phone going off, the doorbell ringing (if you work at home), or any other kind of interruption. There are very few good reasons to respond to your cell phone during a session. (Perhaps, if you knew that the Nobel Peace Prize committee was going to call during that hour, but even so, you would need to warn the client of a possible interruption!). Make sure you have turned off your phone and pager and ask your clients to do so as well. Some clients will balk at that, but you can at least make a strong suggestion, letting them know how counterproductive it can be for their pager to go off when they are deeply relaxed. And there will always be exceptions; a doctor may have his pager on at all times, or a client may have a family member in the hospital and feel uncomfortable about turning off their phone. You have to be reasonable in realizing that not everyone can accommodate your request to leave their phone off.

Practitioners who work at home need to keep the environment as free of interruptions as possible—for example, turn down the phone, put a "Do Not Disturb" sign on the front door, and advise friends not to drop by and family members not to interfere.

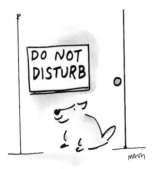

If an interruption is unavoidable (the sink is stopped up, and the plumber is coming), let clients know before the session starts that there may be a brief interruption and that you will make up the time lost. If you know before the appointment time that a session may be interrupted, you can even call clients and forewarn them. Everyone has an occasional emergency—both clients and therapists. If a family member has been involved in an accident or fallen seriously ill, that has to be the priority. If a session is interrupted for such a reason, handle it as quickly and professionally as possible while still being client centered. If you say to the client, "Don't worry about today's session, just get to the hospital to be with your mother. I'll call you later and we'll reschedule, you are truly being client centered and compassionate."

REAL EXPERIENCE

A first-time client arrived very early for her session and had a child of about 5 years old with her. As soon as they entered the office, he walked to the literature rack and started pulling brochures and magazines out and throwing them on the floor. She said nothing to him; I asked him to put them back. There was a bowl of hard candy on the desk, and he turned the bowl upside down. He was shouting every time he opened his mouth, and his mother never acknowledged it or tried to control him in any way. Since she wasn't saying anything to correct him, I told him several times that he had to be quiet because people were getting massage and trying to relax. After a few minutes of his wild behavior, I asked her if someone was coming to pick him up, and she said "No, he's just going to stay with me." At that point, I told her we couldn't allow that, and that she would just have to reschedule her appointment when she could come without him. She said "But I really need this massage!" I replied "So do the other people who are here now in their sessions, and it's not fair to them to have their massage disturbed." She left and didn't come back. I didn't ask her to pay for the canceled session—it was worth the money to get him out of the office and keep him from ruining everyone else's massage. I wasn't trying to be heartless, but I couldn't let him disturb the whole office with his behavior and her lack of concern with it.

—H.W., LMT

Practitioners should do their utmost to see that no one walks in on a session. Clients will be startled by that, no matter who the intruder is. A friend relates:

➤ *One of my most uncomfortable massages was from a woman who worked out of her living room and had a 3-year-old child. Throughout the massage, whenever I opened my eyes, I'd see the curious little girl peeking in. She didn't say anything or actively take her mother's attention, but just having her there took away my privacy.*

Practitioners Avoid Casual Discussion of Treatment or Sessions with Clients Outside Office Boundaries

It's a boundary violation to initiate casual conversation with a client about his or her treatment outside a session. When you see clients in another setting, you may be tempted to talk about their last session: "Is your back still sore?" or "I hope you're feeling better." These may seem like innocent remarks, but when you carry your therapeutic role to another setting, you confuse the boundaries. The safety of your office setting allows clients to relax and show sides of themselves that they might not ordinarily show, both physically and emotionally. Aside from showing their unclothed bodies, they may, for instance, show a more dependent or needy aspect of themselves that isn't usually part of the face they present to the public. When you see clients at the grocery store and say cheerfully, "Hi, how's your back?" you've just, in effect, dragged their naked and vulnerable body into the store—and violated their confidentiality. If *they* initiate the conversation and say "I feel so much better since my massage!" just say "I'm glad I was able to help," and refrain from discussing their issues in public.

When clients see you outside the office and initiate a conversation about the last session or their physical symptoms, it is a great time to practice setting limits. "You broke your toe? Oh my goodness, that's too bad. Give me a call, and let's set up a time when I can see you." Or, as you slowly back away smiling, "Oh, how interesting. We can talk about that next time you come in."

Of course, if clients contact you by phone or e-mail and have questions or concerns about previous sessions or their responses to them, you need to answer their questions and address their concerns. You want to set aside time in your workday to respond to such calls. However, you should avoid talking with clients about treatment concerns at public places or social gatherings, or any time or place outside your office or outside the time you have set aside to answer or receive business calls.

The Internet has opened up so many new areas for boundary complications. Some Internet providers have "instant messaging" features that enable customers to know when another customer is online and then "chat" with him or her. Despite the seeming anonymity of socializing online, Internet boundaries should follow the same guidelines as in-person boundaries. For example, someone may make a post on your personal or business Facebook page, asking if you have an opening at a certain time. Respond with a private message; even though *they* apparently don't mind if everyone knows their business, you shouldn't have a public conversation about it.

Avoid exchanging anything but minimal social greetings with clients outside the office. Also, you don't want to send clients e-mails without their permission. You can put a statement on your intake form such as "Please provide your e-mail address if you would like to be contacted by e-mail for appointment reminders and to receive our monthly newsletter." Always have an unsubscribe option and honor any requests for stopping e-mails.

Practitioners Carefully Safeguard Clients' Rights to Privacy and Confidentiality

Nothing that goes on in your sessions—either what clients say or their physical situation or reactions—should be conveyed to others. You shouldn't give others information about a client without the client's written permission, nor should you repeat anything a client says in a session, no matter how seemingly insignificant. If you are in private practice, the fact that someone is a client should be kept as private as possible. (Situations in which you can make exceptions to confidentiality rules are discussed in Chapter 5.) If you work in a situation where clients will see each other in the reception area, obviously total privacy can't be safeguarded.

The Health Insurance Portability and Accountability Act (HIPAA) sets forth strict confidentiality guidelines that apply to practitioners who use electronic means (faxes and computers) to send information about clients to insurers for billing purposes or who obtain information about clients from medical practitioners.

It is beyond the scope of this book to discuss these guidelines in detail, and practitioners to whom the HIPAA requirements apply should seek more complete guidelines. However, all practitioners need to be aware of procedures for obtaining permission and guarding privacy. HIPAA guidelines may be found at www.hhs.gov/ocr/privacy/index.html.

Obtaining Permission

If you work for yourself, along with getting the client's consent for treatment during the intake process, you should have the client sign a permission form that enables you to obtain information about the client from other health-care practitioners and give information about the client to other health-care practitioners, as needed. If you plan to discuss your clients in supervision or consultation, you should also have written permission from the client to do so. Keep in mind that the client has the right to refuse to give permission. You should also give clients a written statement of your privacy and confidentiality policies, letting them know that you will safeguard all information about them. Ideally, if you work for someone else, that establishment should maintain good policies on confidentiality as outlined in this section and the following one on guarding privacy. However, once you take a job, you may not have control over such policies.

For reasons of their privacy, you or your employer should have clients' permission to call or send e-mail or regular mail to their home or office. Let them know that on some occasions you may need to cancel or change an appointment and ask them how they would like to be contacted. If you are trying to reach a client and must leave a message with someone other than the client or on a shared answering machine, do not identify yourself as that person's massage therapist; just state your name and number and request a return call.

If you send marketing pieces or special offers in the mail, it's best to get written permission from your clients to send them material. Use a form that the client can sign for all of these permissions so that you can keep a clear record of them. If you're keeping client records in a database, you should have an easy method for keeping track of permissions, such as highlighting a client who doesn't wish to receive phone calls at home or work.

Guarding Privacy

It's important that no one else has access to information about your clients without your consent. Keep all information about clients in a password protected file, or if using paper in a locked file or some place that others cannot get into, and keep your online calendar or appointment book and clients' checks out of public view. Staff members such as receptionists also need to know how to keep clients' information private. Unless the client has given written permission for you to speak to their spouse or other family members, you should never divulge information to them, even their appointment time. For all you know, someone who calls claiming that their spouse forgot the day and time of their appointment may actually be an ex-spouse with a restraining order against them who is planning to show up at your office in order to make trouble. It's unlikely, but it could happen. When spouses or domestic partners are both clients, you should not be discussing one with the other. If they've arrived at the same time for appointments with two different therapists, then obviously, one knows the other is there, but you should still refrain from discussing the details of their treatment or other personal matters with them.

Respecting confidentiality also means that arrangements should be made so that people walking by your office door can't overhear the talk during a session. An easy way to block sound is to use a machine that makes white noise. You can also use a solid door, a double door, or a door with soundproofing at the bottom and top. External doors are solid, unlike most standard interior doors, and are helpful for privacy. You may wish to replace your treatment room entrance with one.

Clients Are Unaware of Each Other

Some mental health-care providers who do classic psychotherapy or psychoanalysis arrange their schedules and office entrances and exits so that clients don't see each other. One client leaves from one door at 10 minutes to the hour, and the next one comes in a different door on the hour. The goal is to maintain clients' privacy and cut down on the potential for their imaginings about the therapist's relationship with other clients.

I know of no bodyworkers who separate clients' entrances and exits. Most don't even think of it—or are not in a position to, if they share workspace with other practitioners in a busy office, to schedule clients so that they arrive and leave without seeing each other. While it's a good idea, you're still going to have people who arrive early or take a few minutes extra to leave. You don't know how it will affect one client to see you being warm and friendly as you say goodbye to the previous client at the door; it may mean nothing, but it may stir up the client's insecurity. You can avoid that issue by treating everyone the same—don't gush over one client or discuss any personal matters while another one is sitting there.

A colleague reports:

➤ *Waiting to get a session from a much-loved bodywork teacher, I saw him walk out of his previous session with his arm around his client, chatting in a friendly way. I felt great annoyance and dismay and watched myself spin off into a negative internal monologue: "He doesn't do that with me. He likes that other client better than he likes me. He probably doesn't like me at all."*

Because my colleague had a solid history of trusting that teacher, her reaction didn't last and the situation didn't interfere with the session, but it could have been disruptive. It could have been one of those sessions when the practitioner didn't understand why the client was being "difficult."

If you work alone and you're in the position to arranging your schedule so that clients come and go without bumping into someone else is also considerate of the fact that as they leave your office, they're not always in a frame of mind to deal with other people. They may think their hair looks messy, or they may be so relaxed they're just in a hurry to get home and take a nap, not in a state to want to make polite chitchat.

Depending on your work situation, you may not be able to isolate clients from each other. Keep in mind that the main goal is for clients to be unaware of your professional relationships with other clients. For this reason (and most importantly, for confidentiality), you don't name your clients to each other. Sometimes a client may say "I saw Jack Richards going out the door when I came in. How's he getting along since his wife died?" or some other personal questions. The correct answer is "I can't answer that; I'm bound to abide by confidentiality. But don't worry—that means I won't discuss *you* with anyone, either!" Saying it with a little humor like that will defuse the situation. You don't want the clients to feel like you're scolding them like a parent would scold a misbehaving child.

Even if you don't say another client's name but give information about him or her, it gives the impression that you are loose with client's privacy, and it takes the focus off the present client. Occasionally, it might be reassuring to a client to hear that others have the same kinds of problems. For instance, you could say, "I've noticed that many of my clients seem much more tense during the holidays." However, in deciding whether to make such a comment, you should be motivated by what is best for the client. Create a setting in which each client knows that he or she is the most important person in your (work) life for that hour. If a client sees you warmly hugging another client who is leaving, he or she may be wondering why you don't do the same thing with him or her when *he or she* leaves. Why run the risk of stirring up something that will interfere with the client's trust?

Practitioners Don't Ask Clients to Attend to Their Needs

It's *never* appropriate to ask clients to take care of you—even in the smallest way. A practitioner might be tempted to ask for such care in an obvious way, such as trying to get sympathy about a difficult divorce or asking for advice about a client's area of expertise. Also, practitioners with good intentions may have the misguided idea that it's friendly or somehow helpful to clients to be open with them about personal issues. Actually, it can be a distraction in what is *their* time. What is truly helpful to clients is giving them your full attention, not bringing your personal life

It's never appropriate to ask clients to take care of you—even in the smallest way.

into the session and not asking paying customers to give out emotional support or free advice.

There are subtle ways you may be asking clients to take care of your needs. You might say things such as, "I've had a rough day, I just wish things would get better for me." "I don't like this hot weather," or "I was up so late last night." Even these subtle messages can create problems. Maybe you've had a hard day, but so have they—and they're counting on you to help their day be easier. When they hear something that sounds like you're not up to par that day, it can interfere with their ability to let go and focus on their own experience, and they may fear they're not going to get their money's worth.

Clients are paying you to put aside your personal needs and do what's best for them. Personal revelations from the practitioner can be off-putting. They may begin to see you, in small ways, as needy and inadequate to handle their problems. They may also get the mistaken idea that you want to have a personal relationship with them.

You're not being deceptive when you keep your personal needs out of sessions; it's just good professional manners. You're not arrogantly pretending that you don't have needs; you're simply being appropriate to the professional setting.

Framework with Clients at Different Stages

When is framework important? Although clients may be at different stages in their relationships with us or have particular needs, the importance of framework doesn't change. As the following examples suggest, framework is important to all of our clients.

New Clients

The first appointment is crucial for setting a professional tone. Clients put off by sloppy framework in the first session simply don't come back. There are no second chances to make a first impression. With a regular client, if you are late, have a messy office, or make an inappropriate comment, the client will probably dismiss it as a momentary lapse. But with a new client who can judge you only by that one appointment, such carelessness can imply unprofessionalism, indifference, or incompetence.

Regular Clients

Regular clients get used to their routines, and their hour may feel like a safe haven. Avoid taking clients out of their patterns. If you have to change the framework— move offices or raise fees, for example—be sensitive in presenting those changes. You need to give clients ample notice (a month or two) about major changes. If your employer is in charge of the framework and makes changes, it can be helpful for you to mention to the client that they may have noticed that things are different and then ask them how the change is affecting them.

Emotional Clients

Sometimes, a client who is usually on an even keel has an emotional upset, such as a death in the family or other personal crisis. Being present and sympathetic is all that's required. Avoid the urge to counsel people. All you need to provide is caring, compassionate touch and a safe atmosphere.

It's actually a kindness to your other clients to let go of the emotionally needy client. When we feel wrung out, resentful, or just plain stressed at the end of a session with the emotionally needy client, our next client is not going to get our best work. We have to realize that someone else (maybe a therapist who is an emotionally needy person in his or her own right) will be a good fit for that person when we're not. It's not always going to be in our best interest to try and keep every client who comes in the door.

Mentally Disturbed Clients

If you're working with clients whose internal process is chaotic, you need to be more attentive to external boundaries. This can be difficult because these clients' own sense of boundaries is usually so scattered that they tend not to honor yours. They may want special exceptions, as in the following case:

➤ *A colleague working with a mentally unbalanced woman reported that his limit-setting abilities were challenged when the client requested that he lower her fee, give her a ride to the session, and work only with one specific area, even though the practitioner's methods called for a whole-body approach.*

Some mentally unbalanced clients will be outside your abilities to work with, and you will need advice from a mental health professional to help you refer them on. However, with others, gentle firmness and consistency are enough to settle them down. Sometimes, you may be in the position of having to refuse a referral of a mentally unbalanced person that another health-care provider has referred to you. That has happened to me several times over the years. In one case, a clinical social worker called me about working with a client. As she was describing him, she said that he suffered frequent delusions. I could not feel safe myself in working with them, and while I felt sorry the condition they were in, I did not feel I could take the chance on endangering myself and others who might be in the office working with them.

Another time, a gentleman walked in the door inquiring about massage. I could tell that *something* was wrong with him, and I gently questioned him about his health history. He mentioned several health issues, none of them related to his mental state. I asked him if he would mind telling me if he was on any medication, and immediately recognized one of them as a psychotropic drug. I asked him if he would be comfortable in signing a release for me to speak to his physician, and he did. As soon as I saw the doctor's name on the form, I recognized him as a local psychiatrist. When I spoke to the doctor, he confirmed my hunch that the man was not a good candidate for massage. He stated that among other issues, the man had behavioral problems, and was sometimes prone to sudden violent outbursts. He had been a repeat visitor to the psychiatric ward and at times had to be heavily medicated and restrained.

We all want to help people, but we can't endanger ourselves, our other clients, and coworkers in the process.

Clients Who Are Traumatized or in Pain

Fear and pain make us more sensitive to orderliness and kindness in the environment. Clients who have experienced a good deal of trauma in their lives may be vigilant and watchful, expecting danger at every moment. Clients frightened by chronic physical pain are like wounded animals that have retreated into a corner. Both kinds of clients can be hypersensitive to any perceived imbalance in the therapeutic relationship. Small framework errors or lapses in attention can make them think we are incompetent or indifferent. Such clients are grateful for good boundaries, and we must be hypervigilant in respecting them.

There have been several research studies regarding massage and other complementary therapies as an adjunct therapy for treating veterans and others with posttraumatic stress disorder (PTSD). Many soldiers come home from war with no visible injuries, but emotional distress that is just as serious, if not more so, than having a leg blown off. Veterans with PTSD, victims of violent crimes, and victims of torture are special populations that require more education than most of us get in massage school in order to work safely and effectively with them. We may need to adjust the way we work in order to make the client feel safe. That may mean keeping the overhead light on in the room, when we're used to working in very dim light, and avoiding sudden movements. It may mean using a pillow or doing side-lying work because the face cradle makes them feel claustrophobic. It may mean being sure that their head is facing so they can see the door. Even something as simple as our accidentally dropping the jar of massage cream on the floor could have a dramatic effect on someone with PTSD. If you intend to work with this population, you should seek special training through continuing education.

Clients with Whom You Have Another Relationship

You can be tempted to be careless about framework with people you know: "I don't have to have the room ready—it's only my buddy Bob." You actually need to be *more* crisp with your boundaries in such cases, to help friends with the confusion of switching roles. Dual relationships are discussed thoroughly in Chapter 10.

Clients Who Have Been Sexually Abused

Extra attention to framework is necessary for clients who have been sexually abused. At the same time, because their own boundaries may be confused, they may push the edges—being flirtatious with you or asking for special treatment. To keep your boundaries safe enough for these clients, part of your framework should include supervision from a mental health professional.

Clients who have been sexually abused may also (understandably) have issues with being touched. They may want to keep clothing on. They may be uncomfortable or not want work done in certain areas—and that may not be obvious until you notice them flinching and gritting their teeth. Long ago, a client seemed to be very uncomfortable when I was working her upper arm. I asked her a couple of times if she was okay and she said yes. The next time she returned for massage, she confided that her abusive father had always grabbed her by that arm, and that the memory of that came up when I was working on it. We don't have any way of knowing the horrors that people have been through, unless they share that with us, and we must always be careful and sensitive to body language and client reactions to what we're doing.

Ending the Professional Relationship: Achieving Closure

You want to do your best to end your professional relationship with clients on a positive note. Leaving clients with negative feelings could color how they evaluate their entire time working with you or leave them with bad feelings about the profession in general. On the other hand, we can't take it personally every time a client stops coming. When people feel so much better than they did before they became a massage client, it sometimes goes out of their consciousness that maintaining a regular massage schedule can help keep them feeling good, and they might need a gentle reminder. Sometimes they've just moved, and there's another therapist that's more convenient to them. It may be that they're ill, or their finances are not allowing them to come, or that they've become a caregiver for a sick family member, but if you don't ask, you won't know.

Contacting Clients Who Quit

Sometimes when regular clients suddenly stop making appointments without giving a reason, you may wonder whether to contact them. You may be concerned that you have somehow offended them or made them uncomfortable. Generally, when clients stop coming and you have decided to contact them, it's a good idea to write a note (handwritten, not e-mailed) and say that you've noticed their absence and that you hope they're doing well. If you have reason to believe you've offended them, you can say that you hope that you haven't inadvertently offended or upset them and that you're open to talking about any concerns they might have. A note is less confrontational than a phone call and easier for both practitioner and client to handle. If you work for someone else, you will have to follow their policies about contacting former clients. If you're employing others in your practice, you need to have a policy on that for your own business.

When a regular client stops seeing you abruptly, your decision about what to do may be influenced by your personal feelings. You may, for instance, feel angry, rejected, or just plain disappointed. If you're confused about what to do or say or if you have many feelings about this client leaving, it would be a good time to talk with a trusted teacher or colleague in a confidential setting to help sort out your feelings. You might even consult with a professional who is knowledgeable about interpersonal dynamics—such as a counselor, psychotherapist, or bodyworker who has psychological training—to help you clarify your response to the situation. (Such a consultation wouldn't involve delving into personal issues as you would in psychotherapy. It would only help you with smoothing out issues that get in the way of good relationships with clients.)

Ending Your Practice

If even small changes in framework are disruptive to clients, what is it like for them when you leave town or retire and end your practice? If you terminate with clients carelessly, you may leave them with a bad feeling about the whole experience of working with you, and even affect how they feel about finding another massage therapist.

You want to give clients adequate notice so that they can get used to the idea of their sessions ending and have time to express their feelings, whether those feelings are anger, rejection, gratitude, or some combination. If you are able, 2 months is a good amount of time to give notice. You can send notes to clients who don't come in regularly so that they don't have a rude surprise when they call for an appointment. Also, be prepared with names of other practitioners to whom you can refer them. Be sure it's someone you've visited personally, and try to find someone whose practice is a lot like yours. If your practice is primarily medically-oriented, then referring them to a practitioner who only does relaxation massage is not a good choice, and vice versa.

You should offer to give the clients their record with your SOAP notes to them before closing your practice so that they may pass them on to their new therapist if they desire. Be sure you adhere to state board rules regarding the amount of time you have to keep records. If the client doesn't want his or her file, or you have saved the files of people you haven't seen in a long time, those should be shredded or burned, so as not to compromise confidentiality.

For practitioners too, it's often emotionally difficult to leave; you may be grieving the loss created by the change or feeling guilty, as if you were abandoning your clients. During this time, getting support from trusted teachers or a professional trained in psychological dynamics can help make the transition smoother so that you can more effectively help clients—and yourself—weather the change.

Bending Framework: A Red Flag

A good reason for being consistent with boundaries is that you will be more inclined to notice when you alter them. It's a red flag when you step outside your usual framework. When you bend your professional boundaries, you encourage others to treat you as if you're not a professional.

When boundaries become like Swiss cheese, clients can fall through the holes.

When boundaries become like Swiss cheese, clients can fall through the holes. Les Kertay, clinical psychologist and former chair of the Rolf Institute's ethics committee, says that making special exceptions for clients is always a red flag for practitioners. One of the main ways people get into big trouble with clients (e.g., ethics complaints) or even small trouble (the client doesn't come back or becomes a "difficult" client) is through treating the client as special in some way.

Would it have been hard-hearted not to make an exception for a client in great pain? You want to distinguish between a client who is sincerely in a crisis and a client who has a pattern of being manipulative. That can be a difficult judgment call, but there are often clues. For example, a client may call and say that she is in terrible distress and must be seen right away. If the practitioner says, for instance,

REAL EXPERIENCE

A colleague relates:

There has been only one time in my 20 years of practice when I didn't get paid—and it was a client for whom I had made exception after exception. I allowed my judgment to be clouded for several reasons: she had a large area of scar tissue on her chest and neck from a traumatic childhood injury; she said she was in a great deal of pain, and she was a struggling single mother.

Rushing in to rescue her, I discounted my fee substantially and would see her at times when I didn't usually schedule sessions. She never seemed to get relief from the pain, and that would double my desire to "fix" her. The last time I saw her, I agreed to work on my birthday, although I had planned to take the day off. To make it worse, I was giving her a discount. At the end of the session, she said she didn't have her debit card any checks with her and that she would mail me the fee. That was the last I heard from her. Stiffed on my birthday—it's a lesson I remember. I had created my own disaster by allowing—and even facilitating—the client violating my boundaries.

"I can't see you Sunday, but I have an opening at 10 a.m. on Monday," and the client responds, "Oh, I can't then. That's when I get my hair cut," or needs to take the dog to the vet, or provides another seemingly flimsy response, the client isn't being straightforward. Other clients may describe awful pain and want to be seen immediately, but when the practitioner asks how long they've had the pain, they'll say, "Six years." Their pain may be real, but you may not need to rearrange your schedule to see them right away.

You don't do clients a favor when you let them hook you into ignoring your own framework policies. You also don't need to judge clients who want to be treated in a special way. The client in the case above who didn't pay was simply dealing with a difficult situation in an unhealthy way that she'd learned a long time ago. It was a mistake for the practitioner to continue to treat her in a special way, and it wasn't helpful to the client. People heal best when they have a safe container, and this client never knew where the boundaries were.

If someone has been injured or is in emotional crisis, depending on the circumstances and your schedule, you may want to make an exception for him or her. Special exceptions need to be carefully considered and consistent—but be realistic. If a client calls with the news that they were in a car accident a couple of hours ago and their neck hurts, you don't need to throw caution to the wind by telling them to come in immediately—you need to ask if they've been to see the doctor and suggest that they go there first, if they haven't been examined since the accident. Experienced practitioners develop their own guidelines about what circumstances will warrant bending the standard framework, and they then avoid going outside their own rules. Firm framework saves energy and stress and provides comfort for both practitioner and client.

Framework Matters

What individual clients need to feel safe varies. There are guidelines, such as confidentiality, that are universally part of a professional code. Others may lend themselves to flexibility. For instance, in some cases, because of either the practitioner's personality or the client's, a cluttered treatment room may not make a difference. In other cases, messiness could make a client uncomfortable. The ultimate authority for framework is the client's experience. Does what you do make your clients tense or help them breathe easier?

Maintaining a stable framework also benefits you. An inconsistent framework—variations in how long sessions run or special deals with fees, for instance—is energy consuming for practitioners.

Although you want to be consistent and stable in your framework, experienced practitioners know that total consistency is an ideal rather than a reality. The point is not to become rigidly locked into rules, but to know that framework matters, and to thoughtfully consider the ways you manage the nuts and bolts of your practice.

Questions for Reflection

1. As a prospective client of a somatic practitioner (or other professional), has your decision regarding whether to make an appointment ever been strongly influenced, pro or con, by the practitioner's demeanor during the initial phone conversation? What made the difference?

2. Has the appearance of a manual therapist's office or work environment ever been off-putting for you? What made you uncomfortable?

3. In your work life, have you ever made an exception for a client or customer and then been sorry you did? What happened, and what motivated you to make that exception? What did you learn from that experience?

4. Why do you think we need consistency in this work?

5. Have you ever chosen one professional (or any kind of service person such as a plumber or car mechanic) over another because of their attention to framework details?

thePoint® To learn more about the concepts discussed in this chapter, visit http://thePoint .lww.com/Allen-McIntosh4e

CHAPTER 4

Client–Practitioner Dynamics: Boundaries and the Power Imbalance

For a deeper understanding of the need for good boundaries and framework, we have to take a closer look at our relationships with clients. Often those relationships are more complicated than they appear at first. Much is going on beneath the surface that may seem puzzling and challenging, making it difficult for practitioners to stay clear headed and compassionate.

Clients respond to us in ways we can't always explain—sometimes they touch our hearts, and sometimes they push our buttons. Some clients act as if we're gods, and others seem monumentally unimpressed. Not all clients are going to feel we're the authority; a physician, for example, is probably not going to be subject to the power dynamics that are often at play in the therapist–client relationship, nor are people who are full of their own self-confidence. Some are as open to us as children, while others seem to be wearing a suit of armor. Sometimes we feel drained by clients, and other times, we feel exhilarated by them. Often we don't understand either reaction. It's best to represent yourself honestly as a licensed massage therapist—you don't have to claim to be an "authority."

Transference and Countertransference

Understanding the built-in power differential (defined in Chapter 1) between us and our clients is the key to unraveling the complexities of those relationships. We are more important to our clients than we often realize. When we take on the role of practitioner, it is that role, not necessarily who we are personally, that gives us special authority or power in clients' eyes.

For one thing, the intimacy of the situation may bring up unconscious issues for clients (and, as we will see later, for us as well). On some level, those unconscious factors can tend to make clients feel dependent on us or even like children. Consider the circumstances that we work in: we are clothed, our clients are naked or close to it. We are active, they are relatively passive. What we are doing and why we are doing it are often unclear to them—not because we have not explained it well, but because much of our work defies verbal explanation. Our touch is often nurturing, sometimes probing, but always personal. Also, clients (and practitioners) are often in an altered state of consciousness, a state in which they are less in their thinking minds and more open and vulnerable than they usually are in their day-to-day lives. Add these factors together, and we can begin to appreciate the strong influences going on during sessions.

It's natural for clients to experience us—again, on an unconscious level—as an authority figure. In their minds, we become a little (or a lot) larger than life and more powerful than they are. Everyone has more or less unresolved issues related to parents or authority figures, and clients bring those issues into the session. Because of that, clients may look up to us with far more admiration than they would if they met us in another context. Or they may be more wary of us than they would ordinarily be.

Psychological theory calls the process of how clients react to the power imbalance as **transference**. Old hurts, longings, and conflicts from a client's past relationships with authority figures or important others are unconsciously *transferred* to us in our role as practitioner. For instance, a client who was physically abused as a child may have an unconscious fear of being injured by the large person (and we all look big as we stand over clients) looming over them. Or clients who felt lonely and abandoned as a child may hope for their practitioner to be the all-giving, unconditionally loving parent they wished they'd had.

Transference:
When a client unconsciously projects (transfers) unresolved feelings, needs, and issues—usually from childhood and usually related to parent or other authority figures—onto a practitioner.

How do we know that transference is happening? Clients aren't usually consciously aware of these feelings, so they don't generally talk about them. Instead, we see transference in the ways clients relate to us. For instance, some clients defer to us and never question our judgment, others show adoration or develop crushes, and still others seem to mistrust us for no obvious reason. ("Crush" in this context describes a feeling of admiration for or attraction to a practitioner that is similar to the innocent feelings that a third grader has for his or her favorite teacher. Although there may be a hint of sexual feeling, the client doesn't attempt to act on it.)

What does transference mean to you in your role as a caring practitioner? Transference can happen immediately, the first time a client meets you, and can deepen with an ongoing relationship with a long-term client. Transference is a very common aspect of your relationship with any client, whether a one-time or a regular client.

You will never understand all that is going on inside your clients, and you should not try to be their analyst. But you do need to know that the dynamics of your interactions with clients are more complex than they seem. You also need to know how to help clients feel safe with you in light of these dynamics.

REAL EXPERIENCE

A 50-year-old client related during one of her first sessions that when she was a teenager, her mother had committed suicide. She spoke of it as a matter-of-fact, and said that although it left her in turmoil for many years, that it was now so long ago that she was "over it," but I doubted that, as she often brought it up. She was married to a busy doctor, and they had a son in his 20s who had a lot of emotional problems and still lived at home. He suffered from anxiety attacks and bipolar disorder, and from many things she said, it had been a big strain on the marriage and the family as a whole. She had been a client for several years when her son decided to move away from home. He moved to the coast, enrolled in college, got a part-time job, and she thought everything was going better when her husband suddenly announced that he was leaving her for another woman.

She spent every session talking nonstop about her problems, and it almost seemed like the massage was just a good excuse to come in and talk to someone who would listen to her. She said she appreciated that I just listened to her without passing judgment or trying to give her advice. She even made a joke that I was a lot cheaper than a psychiatrist.

When she missed her standing weekly appointment one morning, I was concerned, but I figured some emergency had arisen when I was unable to get her on the phone. That afternoon, the police came to my office. She had committed suicide, and left notes for several people, including me.

I knew that she had become emotionally dependent on me, as a sympathetic listener and provider of compassionate touch. I've wondered many times, since she died, if I should have referred her to another therapist long ago, when she first started sharing her personal problems with me. I've wondered if there were any signs that I missed that she was thinking of killing herself. I felt guilty in some way when she died, and ended up seeking counseling myself. This experience has taught me to keep myself more detached from my clients...not unfriendly, but on guard against clients who seem to need a counselor worse than they need a massage. That doesn't mean I freak out if a client shares a personal problem, but if they seem too focused on that, I gently steer the conversation in another direction, and if they don't take the hint, I try some active resistance or something else that they have to focus on and participate in, something I didn't really worry about doing before. It was a sad experience, but I learned a lesson from it.

—Anonymous

Positive and Negative Transference

One way to look at transference is in terms of its positive and negative aspects.

Positive Transference

When a client has special affection or adoration or deference toward us, we call it positive transference.

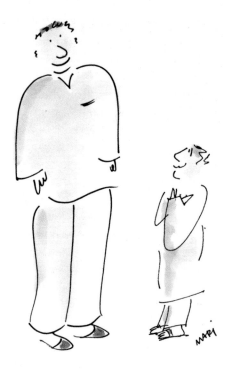

Clients can feel as if they are small and relatively insignificant and we are large and benevolent. We see positive transference most dramatically when clients have innocent crushes on us or are in awe of us and think we are special and wonderful. However, it is usually more subtle, as described under "Signs of Transference" later in this chapter.

Negative Transference

We see negative transference in clients who mistrust us without good reason, who expect us to hurt or criticize them.

Here are two examples of negative transference:

➤ *A new client is nervous and asks an unusual number of questions about the practitioner's qualifications. During the bodywork session, the client pulls back at the slightest hint of discomfort. Later, she reveals that she was physically abused as a child.*

➤ *A male client seems very "controlling," telling the practitioner exactly where and how deep he wants the work to be. He has a hard time relaxing, resists closing his eyes during a session, and is constantly aware of small sounds from the outside. After several sessions, the practitioner learns that the client grew up in a war-torn country and endured constant air raids and fear for his life.*

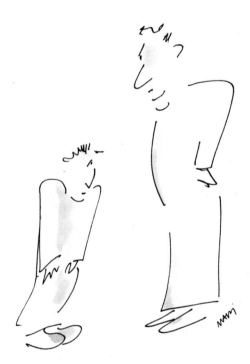

Assuming that the practitioners in these examples provided safe, welcoming spaces and presented themselves as professional and attentive, these clients were not responding to the actual situation in front of them; the danger they were reacting to was in their past, not the present. It's not useful for practitioners to respond with annoyance or dismay when clients seem overly sensitive, try to take charge, or are especially vigilant. Understanding that unconscious fears may motivate such reactions helps us respond with compassion and attentiveness.

With negative transference—when the client is critical of us or doesn't trust us—we sometimes have the feeling of "But I didn't do anything." or "Why does that bother her? It doesn't bother anyone else." Although negativity from the client may feel like a threat or an attack, it is usually no more about us than are positive transference reactions. Human nature being what it is, we often see negative transference as the client's problem, as some kind of character defect, yet we see positive transference as a natural response to our winning personality or exceptional skills.

We can't always know what a client is feeling—or why. In fact, we may misinterpret a client's behavior; clients (and people in general) don't always act the way they feel. A client who feels afraid of us may act defiant. A client who thinks the practitioner is the best thing since sliced bread may act nonchalant. And to make it more complicated, clients often feel both positive and negative transference toward their practitioners. Whatever form the transference takes, be aware that clients are giving extra weight to what we say and do.

Transference, a Normal Process

Transference may sound complex and unusual, but it's actually part of our everyday life even outside our offices. It's normal for any of us to bring the past into our present relationships. In fact, it happens all the time:

➤ *Mary overreacts to her boyfriend's teasing because her father, who teased her, was critical and hurtful in other ways.*

➤ *John feels especially connected to and possessive of a friend who is nurturing to him in a way that John's mother was not.*

These kinds of transference are common in our everyday lives. But they are magnified in a manual therapy session because of the intimacy of the setting, the client's altered state, and the way that the practitioner–client roles mimic those of parent–child.

Once clients connect with us as practitioners, transference just happens. Never mind that our clients are adults or may even be older than we are. Transference isn't a rational process. It's human nature, and we don't need to try to psychoanalyze our clients; we just need to recognize when it's happening, know that we don't need to take it personally, and act professionally. Some well-meaning practitioners will protest, "But I want to be an equal with my clients. I don't want to have any power over them." Although this is a noble idea, transference can't be avoided. The situation isn't a level playing field from the outset. No matter what our good intentions, it's natural that some degree of transference happens.

The minute we take on a client, we acquire a responsibility toward that person. The relationship is unequal, and it is likely to continue that way for as long as we know the client. True, we want to continue to give power back to the client, as appropriate. Ways to do that are discussed later in this chapter.

Countertransference

Practitioners come to bodywork sessions with all their own history, too. Like clients, we're just human; we are in an intimate situation and often in an altered state while we work. In these conditions, practitioners also can lose their objectivity. Old feelings and attitudes can cloud our judgment and interfere with the way we respond to clients. When a practitioner transfers feelings to a client, which belong in the practitioner's past or those that are related to the practitioner's issues, it is called **countertransference**.

> **Countertransference:**
> When a practitioner allows unresolved feelings and personal issues to influence his or her relationship with a client.

Countertransference, like transference, is an unconscious process—usually we're not consciously aware of why we're responding to a client in a certain way. Here are some possible scenarios that show countertransference:

➤ *Massage therapist Martha responds with irritation to a picky, complaining client, who has made many requests. When the client makes one more request, this time for more heat, Martha snaps, "I hope this is the last request you'll make. I can't concentrate on my work." Although Martha's not aware of it, that client reminds her of her chronically complaining mother. Martha may think she's responding as any practitioner would to an annoying client. However, she's actually relating to the client as an angry child would. If Martha stepped back into her professional role, she might realize that the client has a right to ask for alterations that will enhance her comfort.*

➤ *Bodyworker Bill bends over backward for his kindly older client, Robert, who acts as if everything Bill does is wonderful. In Bill's mind, Robert has become the ideal dad he longed for, so he makes extra concessions for Robert, scheduling sessions at times he doesn't usually work and extending credit when he usually requires payment with each session. When Robert doesn't respond as quickly to treatment as Bill wants him to, Bill feels crushed. He doesn't see that he's relating to the client as if he were a child wanting to do anything to please his parent. If Bill was more self-aware and objective, he wouldn't bend his boundaries without good reason, and he wouldn't be discouraged by the normal ups and downs of treatment.*

➤ *When a regular client decides to stop making appointments because his back doesn't hurt anymore, somatic practitioner Sue relates to the event as if the client were the parent who abandoned her. Sue feels angry and rejected rather than having the healthy perspective that she's done such good work that the client is now able to stop seeing her.*

Sometimes, we may experience our own transference the moment we meet a client, before we've even had a chance to get to know them. A client comes in the door and reminds you of your ex-mother-in-law who didn't think you were good enough for her son and constantly made cutting remarks to you, and you take an immediate dislike to her. The poor woman hasn't done a thing wrong or harmed us in any way, and yet, there's that gut reaction—just because she happens to look like someone we have an unpleasant association with! We need to recognize when that's happening, too, and keep it in check where our clients are concerned. If you realize that your professionalism is slipping, discuss the situation with a mentor. If you can't be professional and cordial to a client, refer them to someone else.

REAL EXPERIENCE

When I first started in massage, I worked in an office group practice with several other therapists, and one of my coworkers had a regular client that I thought was very sweet and attractive. He was always friendly when he came in for his massage, and I have to admit I had a little crush on him. If I saw his name in the appointment book, I made sure to take a little more care with my dress and makeup on the day he was coming in. The therapist who usually saw him had an emergency one day just a couple of minutes before he was due to arrive. She knew I was finished for the day and asked if I could stay to let him know what had happened, and to give him the massage if he was agreeable to that. During the massage, I could not stop myself from admiring his body and indulging in a few fantasies. My heart was pounding while I was giving him the massage, and I was actually glad when it was over! I figured I had better never massage him again, no matter what the circumstances were. It was scary for me to realize that I felt that physically attracted to a client, even though he wasn't really *my* client and it was just a one-time massage. A couple of months after I gave him the massage, he moved out of state and never came into the office again. I've had a lot more experience in the years since then (and married and had three children), and it's never been an issue again, but I've never forgotten about it. New therapists who are just starting out need to be hyperaware that it *is* possible to feel attracted to a client, and hyperaware that they should never act on it by being flirtatious (or worse).

—Anonymous

Transference and Countertransference Together

A client's emotional transference-driven response can elicit an emotional countertransference response from the practitioner. As an example, consider that when people feel small and defenseless, they may act angry and critical. A client who feels small and defenseless may react with anger or pickiness, and the practitioner, who then also feels small and defenseless, may react with irritation and defensiveness. Both the client and the practitioner feel threatened and end up acting critical or menacing.

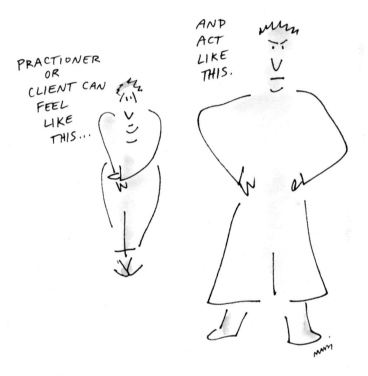

Here's an example:

➤ *Both client and practitioner are perfectionists—both believe that they never measured up to their parents' expectations, and both still carry that insecurity. The practitioner, meaning to give information and sympathy, says to the client, "Boy, you're tight in your upper back." The client hears it as a parental criticism of his ability to take care of himself and responds with an irritated, "That's what you're supposed to help me with!" The practitioner hears that as a criticism of her professional skills and mumbles an exasperated, "I'm doing the best I can."*

A more therapeutic response from the practitioner might be to say cheerfully, "You're right—it *is* what I'm supposed to do! I meant to say that it looks like you've been under a good deal of stress."

Signs of Transference

There are various ways that we can tell that positive or negative transference is in play.

Clients' Passivity

One sign that clients have promoted us to an elevated status is that, in general, clients rarely express their unhappiness with something we're doing, and they often agree to something they don't really want to do. They may tell us, for instance, that they are fine lying in a position that is actually making their neck

---

REAL EXPERIENCE

The first time I was criticized by a client, I was so shocked, I am afraid I didn't respond appropriately. I did in fact take it very personally. It was a first-time client, and she didn't complain while she was on the table. I had checked in regarding pressure a couple of times, and other than answering me that it was fine, she didn't say anything during the massage. After she came out of the treatment room, I asked "How do you feel now?" and she said "I've had better massage." I'm sure, in retrospect, it wasn't so much what I said, but the tone of voice I said it in, because I immediately got defensive and all I could say was "What was wrong with it?" She proceeded to tell me her daughter was a massage therapist in another state, had in fact purchased the gift certificate she was redeeming, and that her daughter gave a much better massage than I had just given her. I said "Don't you think you might be a little prejudiced?" She said "No, I'm not!" and huffed out the door, and she never came back. I know I overreacted and sounded argumentive. I played the whole scene over in my mind for a few days and decided that the occasional unhappy person was bound to come along and that I needed to be nicer in dealing with them instead of getting defensive and snappy. It was a long time before anyone else had a complaint, and I just said "I'm very sorry. I wish you had let me know during the massage that you were uncomfortable with the work on your upper thigh. We can always avoid anything that makes you uncomfortable." *That* person ended up making another appointment and turning into a repeat client.

—Anonymous

hurt. They often don't speak up when we make them uncomfortable, such as when we've set the room temperature too hot, we're talking too much, or even when they think their practitioner has crossed sexual boundaries. If we make them too uncomfortable, they simply don't come back, sometimes without being conscious of the reason. Or they might remain as clients but become what we call "difficult" clients. The sense of powerlessness that usually goes with being a client is especially noticeable when the client is also a peer. I hear many stories from even seasoned practitioners who have had trouble speaking up when getting work on themselves. You would think that, as professionals, we would have no trouble asserting ourselves, but because of the power of the transference, because of what happens when *we* are on the table, we may be as speechless as anyone else. If we feel powerless to question our colleagues, how must our clients feel?

Here are stories told by practitioners who were the client at the time.

➤ *The session ended 20 minutes earlier than usual, but I didn't question it.*

➤ *The gardener was cutting the grass with a loud lawn mower right outside the window, and it was hard to focus, but I didn't say anything.*

➤ *He expressed sexual interest in me during the session. I told him I wasn't interested. He's such a nice guy that I couldn't tell him how disturbing his inappropriate behavior was to me.*

➤ *He was using really sloppy draping. I knew him and knew he didn't have any sexual intentions, but it still felt bad, and I should have said something.*

Practitioners who tell these stories are usually bewildered or embarrassed that they didn't speak up when they were the client. "I know I should have said something," they say apologetically.

Even in the most traumatizing situations—sexual violations—clients rarely assert themselves. There are many stories of a practitioner intentionally or unintentionally crossing a sexual boundary and then, when later confronted, protesting, "But she didn't say anything."

Sometimes power differences are exaggerated by circumstances that either give the practitioner extra authority or make the client more powerless. For instance, cultural perceptions about authority come into play. The authority gap can be greater when a man is working with a woman or when a practitioner is physically much larger than a client. Also, the power difference is exaggerated when a practitioner is a client's teacher or has special status in the community. It can also be heightened if we are working with a client in crisis.

> ➤ *An experienced bodywork client who was having acute back spasms went to see a bodyworker who was esteemed in the community. The client said, "During the session, I felt like what she was doing wasn't right for me, but this woman is 'the best', and I didn't question her. I ended up feeling injured by her work."*

Practitioners who fit into any of these categories may need to take extra care to help their clients feel safe. For example, all of us need to explain what the treatment will involve, get clients' consent before treatment, and let clients know they have the right to refuse any part of the treatment or ask the practitioner to stop. However, practitioners who know the power imbalance is greater than usual will need to be especially alert to signs of discomfort in clients.

The Captive Audience

Positive transference can be so subtle and pervasive that we can take advantage of it without realizing it. For instance, during a session, we may talk on and on about our philosophy of life while the client listens as if to a guru. Just because the client has fallen into the illusion that we are wiser and somehow better than they are doesn't mean that we have to fall in there with them.

It can be appealing to have an attentive audience that defers to us. In the presence of the admiring (or, at least, not overtly complaining) client, we may imagine we have such interesting (in our own perception, anyway) stories to tell or that our opinions and thoughts on just about anything are especially meaningful. When we allow that to happen, we have forgotten that the client is the star of the show, not us.

Clients may put up with practitioner's self-centeredness. Who would risk offending someone who holds the key to helping them? Clients come to us hoping to feel better, and sometimes they are in pain. Who would risk insulting their bodyworker?

When we mistake positive transference for the truth or when we buy into the idea that we are somehow better than the client, we lose our curiosity about the client—and we lose our effectiveness. What does the client want from the session? What pain is the client ready to release? What are the client's strengths and dreams? Clients know more about themselves than we do—sometimes they simply don't know that they know. Our job is to help them find the best in themselves, not to impose our own needs and egos. Don't get caught up in the "I am the healer" syndrome. We don't "heal" anybody. We're here to facilitate them being able to heal, and that's all. Arrogance is not an attractive quality. Making claims that you can "fix" anyone, or that you've helped every person you've ever worked with, is unnecessary. Let your work speak for itself.

Our curiosity and compassion go out the window when we pretend to be all-knowing or when we forget that the session belongs to the client. Even if clients need to put us on a pedestal, we have to find ways to let them know that, although we are competent, we are merely consultants who have certain gifts and training; they are the ones who have the power in their own lives.

Lost Souls

Isn't it okay to have some clients who really like us, clients with whom we have a great connection? The answer depends on another question: Are our sessions with them about us or about them? Are those clients lost souls coming to hear what we have to say, or are we the ones who listen with curiosity and interest to what they bring to a session?

Some clients try hard to please us, and that can feel good. But by basking in the glow of our own egos, we can miss the desperation underneath their efforts to please. Certified Feldenkrais trainer Paul Rubin talks about clients who are at a time in their lives when they feel like "lost souls:" "Many people are at a choice point of 'Do I find myself, or do I find someone I can see as more powerful with whom I can have a dependent relationship?' It's always up to us to guide people back to finding their independence."

It can be natural and therapeutic for clients we see regularly to be dependent and to look up to us to some degree. Certainly, most of us have had times in our lives when we felt like lost souls and we needed someone to depend on ourselves. However, if our practices are full of people who call us after hours or who rely on us to help them make decisions, then we need to take a look at what's going on. Are we getting our own emotional needs met by cultivating dependency in clients? It's not our job to run our clients' lives. As a colleague Janet Zimmerman so aptly put it, "We have to remember that we're just the hired hands."

Sexual Feelings

Crushes are a common form of transference, and it is easy to think that they are about us. They really are not. (Again, we're not talking about clients who are intentionally sexually inappropriate or aggressive with us.) Crushes don't mean that clients want romantic relationships with their practitioners. Rather, the client's unconscious is using the practitioner (in an appropriate, therapeutic way) to deal with deep issues. For instance, they may see in us the good, nurturing parent they wish they'd had. Or maybe the work itself, the softening of tightly held tissue, has helped them get in touch with old longings, and they then think those longings have something to do with us. Our work with such clients, perhaps our acceptance of them, has awakened something in them, but their feelings aren't really about us.

If the client with a crush is of an age and gender we are usually attracted to, the situation can be more dangerous; it may make it easier both to misinterpret the client's intentions and to return the interest. Practitioners who are drawn to doing that should seek outside help to sort it out. It's unethical to take advantage of a client's romantic transference feelings for us.

How to Work with Transference

Many psychotherapists actively work with transference to help clients heal old wounds, learn new patterns of relating, and so forth. Although that is beyond our scope of practice, we can still be therapeutic in our actions. For instance, if a client is (unconsciously) expecting the worst, such as punishment or criticism, then it must surely be helpful for that client if the practitioner's responses are, instead, caring and reasonable. Or with a smitten client, it can be helpful for the practitioner not to soak up the adulation but, instead, to gently give the power back to the client. That and other guidelines for dealing with transference are provided later.

Don't Talk to Clients About Their Transference

The first rule is—and this is one of the rare times the word "rule" is used in this book—don't talk to clients about what you imagine their transference to be. For instance, don't say, "You're just upset with me because you're still mad at your mother" or "You have a crush on me because you need a strong father figure." Avoid psychoanalyzing people. That is not within our scope of practice. Even if you're doing it in your head, don't voice your opinions about it.

For one thing, you don't really know what's causing their behavior. And second, remember that transference is unconscious; the client may not know what you're talking about and may find it confusing or annoying. It can seem patronizing to tell clients your ideas about their motivations. It assumes both that you know more about them than they do and that you have license to talk about psychological dynamics with them. A client coming to us for a relaxing rubdown, a balancing structural integration session, or an injury-related sports massage probably doesn't have an interest in our psychological theories.

CONSIDER THIS

Some clients may have diagnosed, or undiagnosed, issues that you are not aware of, such as bipolar disorder or clinical depression, that they did not feel comfortable putting on the intake form. Some clients may have other mental or emotional issues that are not keeping them from functioning in society, but that may nonetheless be a problem in their lives. We are not psychologists or medical doctors, and must avoid giving advice that we're not qualified to give. Telling someone that they could give up their Prozac if they would just start getting massage twice a week, or use lavender oil, or any other thing is outside our scope of practice and dangerous to the client.

Understand That Transference Isn't Usually About You

It's worth saying this again: "Transference" means the client's reaction is only *superficially* about you. Whether it's adoration or deep mistrust, it's often not really about the practitioner. (Although there's probably a grain of truth behind their reaction—you've done something that pleases or displeases them—their response is out of proportion to the actual event.) Practitioners are mistaken if they think they really are that perfect when clients adore them or that awful when clients are mad at them.

Practitioners are mistaken if they think they really are that perfect when clients adore them or that awful when clients are mad at them.

Clients may want to take care of you, please you, challenge you, or berate you. None of these responses is necessarily about you. The challenge is to keep an even keel and not be swayed by clients' reactions.

Know When Transference Is About You

Knowing the dynamics of transference, however, doesn't give you license to dismiss all clients' complaints or criticisms as simply their old unresolved issues. If you keep getting the same kinds of negative feedback, it probably *is* about you. Understanding transference should make practitioners more respectful of and sensitive to clients.

There's truth in both positive and negative transference, but that truth is usually about your professional self, not your private self. Clients who love you may be responding to the fact that, during your sessions with them, you are caring, concerned, and sensitive to their needs. However, if clients knew you in your personal life, they would have a fuller, more human, and less idealized picture. By the same

---

CONSIDER THIS

Online reviews are a big thing on the Internet. Reading them occasionally can be an education in what people think about you and your business. You'll have the occasional client that makes an unfounded complaint, or a genuine complaint—maybe you were having a bad day and distracted when they came in—but if several complaints are the same, such as "She gave a good massage, but her attitude was arrogant and she talked about herself the whole time," or "He seemed too flirty to me, it wasn't professional," then you need to be doing a thorough and fearless examination of your own behavior and your own motivations, and discuss with a mentor what you can do to make positive changes.

token, a client who has trouble trusting you may be responding to a problem with your professional behavior, not who you are in your private life. For instance, if you are chronically late in starting sessions, clients for whom punctuality is important might see you as an uncaring and inconsiderate person, regardless of whether that is generally true about you.

Keep the Boundaries Extra Clear

Faced with a strong negative or positive transference, your job is to be extra crisp about boundaries and to pay close attention to framework. If the client is already in "transference" love with you, for example, you would not want to accept her invitation to a party or in any way encourage a more social relationship. If the client is already uncomfortable with you, taking even greater care with the therapeutic environment can help her feel safer. The more you keep boundaries clear, the lower the possibility that transference will become destructive to the therapeutic relationship.

Be Respectful

Whether they exhibit crushes or fears, all clients deserve practitioners' respect, not their judgments. We don't know where any of these feelings originate in clients. We don't know what their histories are or what deep aspects have been stirred, and we shouldn't pry into their personal lives. A colleague tells this story:

➤ *A client complained about being poked by my fingernails, and I debated a minute before deciding to do anything about them. I'd just gotten a manicure—lovely red nails—and I'd just seen my favorite teacher, who also had long nails, work without pain to her client. Nevertheless, I decided to file my nails and was glad I did. Later in the session, my client told me that when she was a child, her mother would punish her by actually cutting her skin with her long red fingernails.*

Don't Take Advantage of Clients

Avoid taking advantage of clients' transference even in small ways, such as using them as an easy audience. And of course, practitioners who use the affection that clients have for them for their own advantage—turning current client into a business or romantic partner, for example—are committing the worst kind of ethical violation.

Keep Giving the Power Back

By your behavior, you can let clients know that this is a therapeutic situation—that you aren't an abusive parent *or* a savior and that the power is in their hands.

CONSIDER THIS

If you're going through personal challenges, it can be tempting to talk about them, especially with a client you know well or feel close to, but that's fraught with potential to create a troublesome situation. If you share that you're in financial distress, for example, a client may feel compelled to offer you help in the form of a loan or gift. That creates a different relationship dynamic that you don't need! When we tell a client our problems, he or she may feel like he or she ought to take care of us, but remember, *the client* is paying *us* to take care of them. In all of our dealings with clients, we need to ask ourselves if our actions are in the highest good of the client—and be sure that we are not taking advantage of the therapeutic relationship.

Sometimes you can tell them these things directly with phrases such as, "You're the expert on your own body" or "Please tell me if you want me adjust the pressure, or to stop what I'm doing at any time." That's especially important with new clients, as it sets the tone for the future relationship.

From your first interview, let them know that you are working with them in partnership. Ask them what they want from their work with you and explain your work as carefully as possible so that they know what is being offered to them. Let them know that you won't take it personally if they want changes in the environment or the work itself—for instance, if they want you to turn the heat up or down, adjust the volume of the music, or work more lightly or more deeply. Avoid treating them like children or creating your own agenda for them. Here's an example:

> ➤ *A client comes to a practitioner for a relaxing massage for her sore back. Without asking the client her wishes, the practitioner decides that the client also needs to do exercises at home and sends her home with instructions. The practitioner is then upset when the client returns and has not done her "homework." Think in terms of educating and suggesting rather than imposing and ordering.*

Think in terms of educating and suggesting rather than imposing and ordering.

Signs of Countertransference

Clients aren't the only ones with transference issues; we're just as human as they are. Countertransference happens when practitioners bring unresolved issues and feelings into the session. When you take what a client says or does personally, it is considered countertransference. For instance, if you're constantly disappointed and angry with uncooperative clients, that's a red flag. What you can reasonably expect from clients is some form of payment and that they treat you with respect. As long as they aren't abusively insulting or disrespectful, clients should be free to complain, become enamored of you, improve, not improve, and generally go at their own pace *without your taking it personally*. If you expect certain kinds of validation—that they get better at a certain rate so you can feel like a "good" practitioner or that they praise your work during every session—that is countertransference and is not useful.

The intimacy of bodywork triggers deep emotions and old feelings, and practitioners are as much a part of that unconscious soup as are clients. Practitioners can easily lose their objectivity. Any strong feelings about a client—anger, chronic annoyance, or even love or caring—can signal that you are lost in countertransference. Another common red flag for countertransference is feeling tired or drained when you work with certain clients. Be curious about any negative reactions to clients, and get help with understanding these feelings. If you constantly find yourself being annoyed with a certain client, and you can't get beyond that, it's better to release them and refer them to another practitioner.

What about being fond of your clients? Isn't it natural that you open your heart to your clients? One way to distinguish healthy affection for clients from unhealthy ones is the extent to which they have become "special" to you. Do you give extra attention to what you're wearing if you're seeing them that day? Do you make exceptions for them that you don't for other clients? Do you give them extra time, rearrange your schedule to accommodate them, or let their bills slide? Do you go out of your way to help them with an outside problem? In other words, do you bend your own boundaries for this client?

A colleague relates:

> ➤ *I was attracted to one of my new clients and at first wasn't conscious of it. After a few sessions, I began to have signs of countertransference: I always looked forward to her session with some excitement and felt "high" at the end. I made a point of telling her about upcoming events that might be of interest to her and realized that this was in hopes that I might "accidentally" bump into her. She had a busy work life, and I often came in earlier than I usually do to accommodate her. After I became aware of what I was doing, I discussed the attraction with a respected teacher and was able to regain my balance with this client.*

If you imagine that you are the only one who can truly understand or help a particular client, you are headed for trouble. If you see yourself as "rescuing" a poor, helpless client, that's a red flag too.

As for negative countertransference, aren't some people just annoying? Perhaps. But it also could be that another practitioner would find them endearing, or it

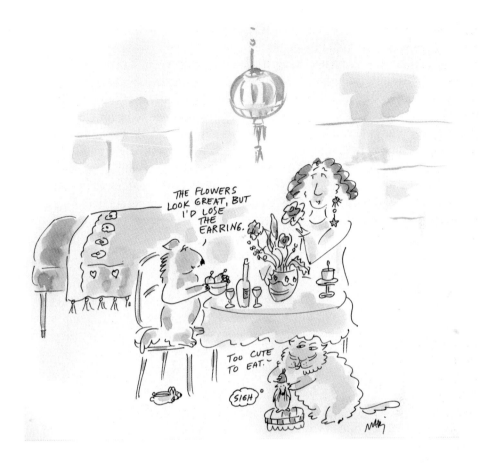

CONSIDER THIS

Many massage therapists get into the profession because they are at heart caring people who like to help others. Our job as professional massage therapists is to help people—with their aches and pains and stress—but not the *cause* of their stress. It's not our job to try to help them with their family problems, relationship problems, financial problems, or any other personal problems. The responsibility for keeping the therapeutic relationship on a professional level is ours. Getting too caught up in the personal problems of our clients can lead to lapses in judgment, which can compromise that balance between showing compassion and being too emotionally involved.

could be that your "annoying client" is simply anxious or even responding to your careless framework. Do you think a particular client got up that morning with the intention of irritating you and making your day seem longer? Or do you sense that

It's easy to be caring with an appreciative client; picky clients are the true test of our compassion.

that is generally the way he or she copes with situations that are difficult for him or her?

Clients who seem difficult or demanding are often trying to mask their underlying fear, neediness, or confusion. The helpful response to these clients is actually just the opposite of our natural inclination. Most of us would be naturally inclined to be impatient and have a "get-over-it" attitude with such a client. However, to really settle this client down, we can respond with attentiveness and concern, for instance, to ask for extra feedback about whether they are comfortable—how's the room temperature, do they want a deeper or lighter pressure, or what else do they need to help them relax? It's easy to be caring with an appreciative client; picky clients are the true test of our compassion.

How to Work with Countertransference

Countertransference happens constantly. It's not a question of "if," but rather of when and how it arises and what kind of people you most easily overreact to. And after you think you've got your inner responses to clients figured out, someone walks through the door who turns you upside down and makes you wonder why you feel mad, fascinated, or exhausted. Working with your own transference (which is called countertransference) is an ongoing learning process.

Notice When You Make Exceptions

As discussed earlier, one of the best ways to know when you are acting out of countertransference is to notice when you want to go outside your usual boundaries or change the usual structure of your sessions. When you come in an hour earlier than usual for a client, or take an appointment on your day off in order to accommodate someone, are you responding to a real need? Or are you accommodating him because you feel too intimidated, guilty, or perhaps charmed to ask the client to fit into your schedule? Paying attention to framework and boundaries provides safety for you because countertransference just naturally happens. We're all humans and always have unresolved issues, old wounds, and insecurities that color our judgments.

Get Outside Help

After you have identified your own countertransference, you can figure out how best to work with it. Sometimes just being aware of it is enough to overcome it. However, other times, you need to get outside help with both recognizing it and learning how to turn those feelings into a better understanding of the client and of yourself. A good way to learn how to recognize when a client hooks you is to consult with a professional trained in psychological dynamics—a counselor or psychotherapist, for instance. Such consultation can help illuminate your countertransference and deal with your feelings related to your clients' transference.

➤ *A practitioner found herself unusually annoyed with a client—a woman who was slightly older than the practitioner and who seemed sweet but passive. In talking with her consultant, the practitioner realized that the client reminded her of her mother's passivity, which often angered her. Once she realized that her feelings were related more to her mother than to her client, she was able to let go of her annoyance.*

Talking over your responses to clients with a mentor or consultant can help you gain the objectivity you need to be skilled in your client relationships. Some practitioners prefer having an ongoing relationship with a consultant for support and help with identifying their strengths and weaknesses in relationships with clients. A consultant can help you know, for instance, when it may be appropriate to refer a client to someone else. If you've done your best to find compassion for a client but are still constantly irritated, you're not helping such a client by continuing to work with him or her. Likewise, if you've discussed your feelings of attraction to a client and those feelings are still intruding into a session, you need to refer that client to another practitioner. It is against professional ethics to work with clients toward whom you have strong feelings of either attraction or repulsion.

Practitioners who regularly consult with professional counselors or bodyworkers trained in psychological dynamics find that it helps them sort out these issues and makes their jobs easier. Strong positive or negative feelings about a client are red flags. Getting outside help can turn those annoyances or infatuations into solid learning experiences.

Hearts and Minds

Giving and receiving bodywork can both touch our hearts and cloud our minds. Bodywork may bring up unconscious material—for our clients as well as ourselves—that can interfere with the therapeutic relationship. Clients get mad at us, clients fall in love with us, and we get irritated or love them back. Our role is to sort out those feelings in a way that empowers and benefits our clients. Our job is to do our best to keep our own issues from intruding into the therapeutic process.

Clear boundaries and a sturdy framework help both parties handle their transference and countertransference reactions. They orient us and bring clarity to the murkiness that arises from unresolved personal history. When we strive to be consistent and even handed, we can identify our red flags more quickly and get help when heading down the wrong path. It takes careful thought, training, and determination not to let the power imbalance inherent in the therapeutic relationship throw us off.

Appreciating the power of transference and countertransference is the key to understanding why we need to take care with boundaries and framework. In fact, the power imbalance between client and practitioner is the reason for most professional rules of ethics. Without an understanding of those dynamics, ethical and boundary guidelines can seem like arbitrary dictates rather than necessary structure.

Questions for Reflection

1. Think of a situation when you were the client of a manual therapist (or other practitioner) when the practitioner was doing something that you didn't agree with or that was making you uncomfortable. Did you question the practitioner at the time or assert yourself? If you did assert yourself, did something that the practitioner said or did make it easy for you to do so? If you didn't, what could he or she have done to make it easier?

2. As an adult, have you ever had a crush on someone who was in a professional role with you? How did the professional handle it? Do you think they were aware of it? What was helpful or not helpful in the way the professional responded to your crush?

3. Have you ever felt small or helpless with an authority figure or a practitioner and then acted "big" and angry? What other ways do you react in the presence of an authority figure? Did you feel threatened?

4. Can you think of a recent time in your everyday life when your response to someone may have come from old perceptions or patterns (transference) rather than the reality of the moment?

5. Have you ever had a manual therapist or practitioner use you as a captive audience? How did you feel? If you didn't like it, did you express that at the time? Did you return to that person, or find someone else to work with?

thePoint To learn more about the concepts discussed in this chapter, visit http://thePoint .lww.com/Allen-McIntosh4e

CHAPTER 5

Ethical Boundaries: From Theory to Practice

We can look for simple answers about ethics—what are the rules, and how do we stay out of trouble? The state boards that regulate massage spell out ethical behavior; note that not every state has a "massage board"; in some states, massage regulation falls under the domain of another board. The massage associations, such as ABMP (Associated Bodywork & Massage Professionals), AMTA (American Massage Therapy Association), and the NCBTMB (National Certification Board for Therapeutic Massage & Bodywork), all have a Code of Ethics. Some massage schools even have their own code. However, there are few black-and-white absolutes to which we can cling. To make wise decisions, we usually have to thread our way through the gray and uncertain areas of the therapeutic relationship with all its details and nuances, its transference and countertransference, and many other boundary issues. Also, to decide the "right" thing to do, we have to consider not only the details of the particular situation, but also the broader picture of how an action will affect our clients, ourselves, our own reputation, and the reputation of our profession.

Ethical Questions

The following questions will help you determine whether an action may lead you down the wrong path. They can help you avoid harm to clients, to your relationship with clients, and to your reputation and the reputation of the profession.

- Would this action take advantage of the power, affection, or goodwill that clients give me because of my role (transference)?
- Would it violate the client's privacy or confidentiality?
- Would it create a dual relationship (a relationship with the client outside that of client and practitioner) and, therefore, make the professional relationship less clear?

- Would it exceed the boundaries of the original implied contract—going beyond either my area of expertise or what the client has agreed on?
- Would it be an exception to my usual policies?
- Regardless of how an action appears to me or my client, would it look inappropriate to others?
- Would the action be disrespectful of the client?

It may be obvious why some of these questions are included and less apparent why others are. Let's take a closer look at these questions, grouped by their ethical intentions.

Protecting Clients' Vulnerability

- Would this action take advantage of the power, esteem, or goodwill that clients give you because of your role (transference)?
- Does it violate the client's privacy, confidentiality, or any other boundaries?

Most ethical standards are aimed at keeping practitioners from taking advantage of the power difference between them and their clients—using a client's affection and goodwill to benefit themselves personally.

Most ethical standards are aimed at keeping practitioners from taking advantage of the power difference between them and their clients—using a client's affection and goodwill to benefit themselves personally.

Respecting clients' privacy and confidentiality is also a central part of what it means to be professional and to be sensitive to a client's vulnerability.

You can overstep boundaries in small ways—for instance, taking advantage of transference by talking too much during a session, or breaching confidentiality by advising someone who has referred a client that the client has made an appointment. Such actions are not usually intentionally unethical; however, the more disciplined you are in honoring the boundaries of transference and confidentiality in even small ways, the less likely you are to err in more serious ways.

Problems arise if you work for an employer who does not honor clients' confidentiality or respect clients' vulnerability. For instance, there may be spas where the owner may allow and even participate in gossip about clients. And some employers ask their massage therapists to take advantage of their relationship with clients by pushing them to buy retail products. Working with these problems will be discussed later in the chapter.

Keeping Small Boundary Mistakes from Leading to Big Problems

- Would this action create a dual relationship and, therefore, make the professional relationship less clear?

- Would it exceed the boundaries of the original implied contract—going beyond either your area of expertise or what the client has agreed on?
- Would it be an exception to your usual policies?

Significant ethical mistakes rarely come out of the blue. These questions relate to the fact that the more you bend boundaries, the more likely you are to get into serious ethical problems. Many boundary transgressions, such as having dual relationships with clients, aren't necessarily unethical by themselves, but they can become bigger problems if you make a habit of doing them without being alert to the difficulties.

➤ *A massage therapist who often socialized with her clients had a hard time keeping her roles straight. One of the clients she socialized with had told the massage therapist during a session that she had multiple sclerosis (MS) and wanted to keep it a secret. However, one day, another friend was criticizing that client and the massage therapist said, "Don't be so hard on her. She has MS." The client with MS found out about the confidentiality violation and, understandably outraged, filed an ethics complaint against the therapist with her professional association. A breach of confidentiality that would have been disturbing enough had it simply occurred between friends became a violation for which there were serious professional consequences for the massage therapist.*

Avoiding the Appearance of Inappropriateness or Impropriety

- Regardless of how an action appears to you or your client, would it look inappropriate to others?

"Impropriety" may sound like a prim and proper word to the often free-spirited members of this profession. As long as you know you're a good, conscientious professional, you may not want to concern yourself with how something looks to an outsider or, in effect, what the neighbors think. However, you can't ignore the fact that massage continues to be linked in the public's mind to sexual services, and those therapists who wind up in the news accused of sexual impropriety make it harder for the rest of us. Although it's unfortunate that our culture often equates nudity and touch with sexual behavior, that's the reality that you have to live with. It's not fair that the manual therapy profession is sometimes misjudged or that good professionals may have to contend with offensive assumptions, but if you want to help your own reputation and that of the profession, it's best to be cautious.

Consider these statements from well-meaning massage therapists:

➤ *I tell my clients that as long as they're comfortable with it, they don't have to be draped.*

> *I'm interested in dating Bob, so I invited him to come to my office and get a free massage. Since it's free, it doesn't affect my professional image.*

You can imagine how these situations could have a negative effect on the reputation of both the professional and the profession. Suppose a prospective client heard that a massage therapist doesn't require draping. It could color this person's opinion of the massage therapist and, if they weren't familiar with the fact that draping is supposed to be a standard protocol of massage, could color their opinion about all massage therapists.

In the second example, bringing a social and possible sexual element into your work and into your office—off hours or not—is a bad idea. It can give the client or anyone who hears about it the idea that you regularly mix your romantic life with your work.

You should not give people any room for their imaginations to run away with them. Maybe an action seems innocent to you and to the client involved, but how will it look to the public? Your colleagues won't appreciate it if you lower the reputation of massage therapy and bodywork in the community. It means they will have the indignity of fielding many more phone calls from prospective clients who expect sexual services; they will have the annoyance and perhaps danger of many more clients who arrive in their offices anticipating sexual relief; and they will have to endure more rolling of eyes when they tell others what they do for a living. Why risk offending colleagues and promoting harmful misconceptions about the profession?

Behave in such a manner that your friends and colleagues would feel comfortable sending you both their elderly aunt and their teenage son or daughter.

Sometimes, even seemingly innocent actions can give a client the wrong impression. For example, some massage therapists are "huggers." While hugging a client you've been seeing for 10 years is not going to be misconstrued, a client that you've only just met could get the wrong idea, or alternatively, just feel uncomfortable with such an action.

None of us work in a vacuum. Whether practitioners belong to a professional association or not, their behavior reflects on the profession and the other practitioners in their community. It's safest to be above reproach. Behave in such a manner that your friends and colleagues would feel comfortable sending you both their elderly aunt and their teenage son or daughter.

What Happens if You're Accused of Sexual Impropriety

If a client makes a complaint to your state board alleging sexual impropriety—or any other complaint—it can be a disaster. I served for 5 years on our state board and was present for many disciplinary hearings, and have also attended hearings in

REAL EXPERIENCE

My husband and I went out to celebrate our anniversary, and after dinner in a nice restaurant that was in a neighboring town, we decided to go dancing. We went to a club we had never been to. At the end of the bar, there was a woman in a bikini offering chair massage—and throwing back tequila shots while she was doing it. I was so shocked; all I could do was stare. Men were lined up waiting their turn. I was shocked again a couple of weeks later when I attended a continuing education class, and she was in it! When people were introducing themselves, she just told her name and said she did onsite massage. When the class took a break, I walked over and asked her if she was the same woman I had seen doing chair massage in the bar. She said she was. I said "Don't you think that's sending people the wrong message about massage?" She laughed and said "I usually make at least $300 a night in tips. I couldn't care less what kind of message it's sending." Then in a snide voice, she said "How much do *you* make?" I didn't see any point in arguing with her. We're in an unregulated state where there's not even a massage board to report her to. I've never been back to the club to see if she's still there, but I've always wondered if the legitimate massage therapists in her town had a hard time with people because of it. I think we do reflect on each other, and it disturbs me to think that the people who see her in the club think this is an honest representation of massage.

—Anonymous MT

some other states. Disciplinary hearings are open to the public. I have encouraged massage school owners and program directors to take massage therapy students on a field trip to their state board to observe disciplinary hearings, in the hope that it might get the message across that this is never a good experience, even if you're innocent.

The fact is, most things that a therapist is accused of take place in the privacy of the massage room, where there are no witnesses, only the two parties directly involved. It's a he said/she said situation. Both parties (the accused and the accuser) have the right to bring an attorney and character witnesses to the hearing if they desire. The board's attorney will be present, and may question both parties, and any character witnesses present. Each party may ask questions of the other, in most states.

A regulatory board hearing is not a court of law, and is allowed more leeway than what takes place in a court of law. I was shocked, at my first hearing as a board member, when the woman accusing a male therapist of sexually molesting her produced a letter from another woman claiming that he had done the same to her. I objected on the grounds that we had no way of knowing if the letter was legitimate and that it was hearsay, and the board's attorney stated "This is not a court of law. Hearsay is allowed here. It is not allowed as the primary evidence for an accusation, but it is allowed as corroborating evidence."

The similarity to a court of law is that the accused has the right to face the accuser. Anonymous complaints do not result in action being taken against a massage therapist, as there is no way to investigate them; however, if there were multiple anonymous complaints received about a therapist, the board may take action, such as sending an undercover investigator in as a client.

After the evidence has been presented at the disciplinary hearing, the board members will usually go into private session to discuss the case. It all comes down to whom they believe made the more credible witness, and the majority rules. That means in a 10-member board, 6 of them have to agree on whether the therapist is innocent or guilty. It does not have to be a unanimous vote. During my time on the board, there were several times when I disagreed with the majority, but that's the way it works. I was convinced, during my tenure of having to sit through disciplinary hearings, that some people were found guilty who did not deserve to be, and that some people who should have been found guilty were turned loose on the public to commit another offense. It is an imperfect system, but again, as there are usually no witnesses, it's the only system we have.

Being found guilty can mean permanent loss of license or temporary suspension of it, a probationary period, paying a fine, being ordered to attend additional ethics and/or other continuing education classes, being ordered to attend a class such as anger management or getting substance abuse treatment, or any combination of the above. In most states, the outcome of the complaint will be listed on the board's website. The client's name will not be revealed, but the listing will say something like "John Smith, License Revoked 01/13/2016, call for details." The Federation of State Massage Therapy Boards also maintains a disciplinary database contributed to by the member states, so that a person who loses a license in one state can't just go to the next state and get one.

In some serious cases, the client may also file a criminal complaint, and/or institute a civil lawsuit. Being accused is emotionally distressing; it affects your reputation and your income. Even if you are found innocent, the fact that it may have gotten publicity can ruin your chances at getting employment or getting clients, if you're self-employed. It's a very serious matter.

Respecting Clients' Dignity

- Would the action be disrespectful of the client?
Consider these cases:

➤ *The client of a deep tissue bodyworker left a message on the bodyworker's answering machine after his first session, complaining that the pain in his back had gotten worse since the session. The bodyworker decided that the client must be a chronic complainer and a nuisance and never returned his call.*

➤ *A massage therapist's client complained that she still had discomfort in her knees even though she had been coming for regular massages for weeks. The practitioner curtly responded, "If you'd lose some weight and get off the sofa and exercise, you might feel a lot better."*

Generally, it's easy to treat clients with respect if they are appreciative and pleasant. Clients such as the two mentioned earlier, who complain or who are demanding (in your perception), are the ones who are most likely to try your patience and test your professional diplomacy. As a professional, you are obligated to respond to complaints with kindness or at least with civility. Even if a client is being abusive, it's unethical for practitioners to be rude, insulting, or unresponsive.

Clients don't have a right to be personally insulting, call you names, or use harsh or vulgar language. (Of course, they also don't have a right to be physically threatening or sexually inappropriate.) However, they do have a right to complain about your work or question your professional knowledge, and you want to be able to respond to their concerns with care and objectivity. Complainers usually need education and reassurance. Depending on the situation, the client whose back was still hurting might need to hear, for instance, that it often takes a day or two before a client feels relief from pain. Or with the client whose knees still hurt, you could let her know you're on her side: "I'm sorry you're still having discomfort. Massage therapy often relieves joint pain, and I was hoping that it would help you."

Maintaining a good professional relationship with your clients also goes a long way toward keeping you out of major trouble. A small complaint handled poorly can balloon into a big problem; angry clients sometimes air their grievances in the community or, at the extreme, take them to your professional association. Many clients also leave reviews of businesses on the Internet these days. There's the occasional complainer in every crowd, but a few bad reviews can really make a negative impact on your business—just like glowing reviews can make a positive difference. If several people make the same complaint, such as "she didn't listen to me, and she talked too much" or "his office wasn't very clean," then you need to pay attention to that.

Judgment Calls

We want to follow the standards of our state and national associations, but sometimes those standards are so generalized that it's difficult to know what they mean in practice. The goal is to learn how to make smart and ethical choices under any circumstance.

In any practice, certain situations require judgment calls on the part of practitioners who want to protect their clients, the profession, and their own reputations.

Keeping in mind the questions and considerations already discussed, here are some examples of how to make good choices and judgment calls.

Sexual Relationships

The Ethical Standard

There's no gray area here; it is unethical to have a sexual relationship with a current client. With an ex-client, it is unethical to use the affection, power, or intimacy of the client–practitioner relationship to create a sexual relationship. It is also unethical to sexualize the relationship with a client by dressing seductively, flirting, or making remarks that could be construed as sexual.

Judgment Calls

Consider the following:

➤ *You run into someone you dated for a couple of years in college, whom you had a sexual relationship with. You haven't seen him in over 20 years and he has moved back to the area. As you are chatting, it comes out that you're both single. He asks what you do for a living, and when you say you're a massage therapist, he raises his eyebrows and says he wants to make an appointment. Do you make the appointment?*

➤ *At a party, you are talking with someone you have just met, someone you find attractive. The person learns that you are a bodyworker (or massage therapist or movement teacher) and wants to make an appointment. Do you make the appointment?*

➤ *You have been working with a client for several months, and you realize that you are starting to feel sexually attracted to him or her. What do you do?*

Everyone should know that the absolute rule is not to date or have sexual relations with a client, but what about sexual attractions? The answer depends, for one thing, on how attracted you are:

- Is it just a passing thought?
- Is there a spark of sexual connection between you?
- Are you often aware of being sexually attracted to another person, or is this a rare feeling, so that the attraction takes on greater meaning?
- Are you feeling emotionally off-balance or needy, so that you might be more than usually tempted to act on an attraction?

- Are you feeling particularly open to a new attraction, even though you are married or in a relationship?
- Has it been your experience that you can be mildly attracted to a client without it interfering with your work?

You have to know yourself and your limitations. Sessions should always focus on the client and not on your personal needs. If you have strong romantic or sexual feelings about a client, the feelings usually intrude into the professional relationship. A strong attraction is a good issue to take to a consultant or respected teacher for discussion.

You should also consider the effect of transference. The decision to become someone's practitioner shouldn't be made casually. When someone becomes a client (and often before he or she arrives on the table), transference begins and feelings are heightened on both sides. In the client's eyes, you have already started to become a little larger than life—the compassionate caregiver, the heroic reliever of pain, or the nurturing parent figure. Under these circumstances, clients are not as free to refuse romantic invitations. It's unethical to take advantage of this vulnerability.

Once someone becomes a client, you may never be able to have a normal social relationship with that person. The effects of transference can be too deep. Once you become a person's practitioner, you have limited the relationship. Most associations' ethics standards require that practitioners wait at least 6 months before dating an ex-client. Regardless of the number of months that have passed, practitioners dating an ex-client could be a cause for concern and perhaps scrutiny in their professional circles. You're better off deciding from the beginning whether a relationship will be professional or social.

There are also varying levels of social relationships, and that may be magnified if you live in a rural area or small town. For example, in those situations, you may attend the same church, eat at the same restaurants, and shop in the same stores. You're going to run into clients; it's unavoidable. If you walk into the local diner to grab lunch, find it crowded, and a client invites you to share his or her table, that may not be a big deal; if the same client were to invite you for an intimate dinner date, that's a different thing altogether. A client may invite you to the annual barbecue at his or her ranch; he or she tells you that they do it every year and expect about 200 guests. That kind of situation isn't apt to cause trouble in the therapeutic relationship, but attending a dinner at their home where you're the only guest, or there are only a few other people present, is trickier.

Let's look back at the three examples. In the first example, the course of action should be clear. This is someone you have already had sex with, albeit a long time ago. He's single, you're single; old feelings may come up. In fact, you used to give him massage when you were an item, although you hadn't been to massage school yet and weren't a professional therapist. It's best not to go there. If you want to see him socially, you can let that be known, but you may need to say something like

"I'd rather get together for a burger. If you really want a massage, I think it would be best if I refer you to a friend of mine. I like to keep business and personal relationships separate."

In the second situation, how do you decide whether to make the appointment? To start with, it's never a good idea to make an appointment or do business at a party. Just offer the person your business card. That would also give you time to sort out your feelings, either on your own or with outside help. If you know you're not in danger of acting on your sexual attraction, you can take the person as a client, knowing that you are thereby eliminating the possibility of having a sexual relationship with him while he is a client and possibly forever. If you're not sure whether you want to exclude that possibility, it's smart to buy time. For instance, when the person calls, you can simply say you don't have any appointments available and tell him or her to call back after a certain time. Given enough time, you can find your ethical bearings and decide whether to take that person as a client.

In the third situation, in which the practitioner becomes attracted to someone who is already a client, it's probably best to seek out help before making a decision about whether to continue to work with that client. As previously noted, any time you have strong feelings about a client, whether it's strong attraction or strong dislike, it's a good idea to talk with someone trained in psychological dynamics to help you sort it out. If you come to understand the reasons for the attraction, the feelings may dissipate. If they don't, then you probably need to stop working with the client. Any tricky situation calls for a careful examination of the strength and motivation of your feelings, and careful consideration of what is best for that particular client. Such a judgment call can best be made with outside help. Sexual attraction, infatuation, and yes—true love—can all cloud professional judgment.

Negative Judgments

The Ethical Standard

We owe clients our care and attention. We may not connect with a person right away, but if we can't imagine ever having a caring attitude toward a particular client, we shouldn't work with him or her. We need to be on the alert for anything that interferes with our ability to touch a client in a respectful, nonjudgmental way. We are not just touching bodies—we're touching spirits.

Judgment Calls

➤ *Your new client reveals that he belongs to a group that offends your belief system. (e.g., he is a member of the National Rifle Association, a gay rights advocate, pro-choice or he belongs to any group about whom you have general prejudgments—prejudice).*

➤ *Your client does something you find very annoying. For example, she talks constantly, or never talks, has a whiny voice, or talks very loudly. You find yourself dreading her sessions.*

Everyone prejudges other people. It's common for people to make snap judgments based on how people look, the way they dress, or their beliefs. No one is completely untouched by negative attitudes about groups of people that they may have been taught as children—whether by the family, the community, or society at large. In addition, everyone has personal likes and dislikes. The question is how much these negative feelings interfere with your work.

Working with people you don't care for can seriously compromise the safety of the therapeutic environment. You may be inclined to be late, to be less than present, to tune them out, to shortchange them on time, or to lack compassion. Practitioners cannot totally hide their personal feelings from clients. What client wants to be touched by uncaring hands?

We also need to consider that we may be getting our exercise jumping to conclusions about people. Maybe you saw the bumper sticker from an organization you find morally reprehensible on a new client's car when he pulled in (and immediately formed a negative opinion of them)...and then you found out that he had car trouble and borrowed his sister's car. Or maybe you saw the initials "KKK" tattooed on a client—and then found out it is his daughter's initials.

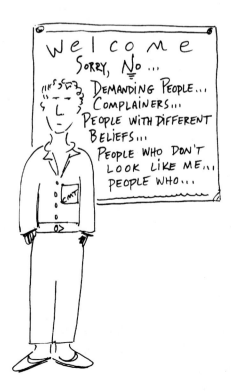

Regarding the first example of a client who belongs to a group that you have judgments about, you want to decide what is best for the client. You must first be honest with yourself about your own prejudices. If you have a thought such as, "Uh oh, here's one of those kinds of people. They are all so lazy/immoral/rigid," do you believe the statement to be true? Or do you recognize it for what it is—a stereotype that may or may not be true for the individual in front of you? As professionals, we are obligated to come to our sessions with an open mind, and opening our minds usually takes some effort. The fact that we may personally know a member of the group who is lazy/immoral/rigid doesn't mean everyone in the group shares those characteristics.

The same holds true for a client you may find annoying or dislike for no good reason—the client isn't being abusive or disrespectful. You have to try to find something in you that connects with that person, something you can open your heart to.

If soul searching doesn't work and your negative feelings are so intense that you can't find compassion for a client, then you need to suggest that the client see someone else. However, even if you refer that client on, once you have identified your own feelings of prejudice or personal dislike, then you are obligated to find a way to work through those feelings, perhaps with the help of a mentor or consultant. If you work for someone else and your employer does not allow you to be selective, then you have to get help with keeping your negative feelings out of the session. (Gritting your teeth doesn't work.)

If you are in private practice and have the freedom to be selective, you can make it clear during the initial conversation with a client that either party can bow out at any time. Nan Narboe, a psychotherapist who consults with massage therapists and bodyworkers, suggests one way to make it easier:

> ➤ *When you make the first appointment, tell your prospective client that the first few sessions will allow the client to decide whether she or he can effectively work with you and also allow you to decide whether your work is the most effective for this client. If you decide that you should not continue working with the client, you can say, "I don't think my work will be as beneficial for you as X or Y" (other methods or other practitioners).*

Taking Financial Advantage of a Client

The Ethical Standard

It is unethical to use the privilege of the client–practitioner relationship to profit financially beyond our fee-for-service charges. It is not ethical to exploit the relationship by using it to influence the client to buy a product or service or to make any investment.

Judgment Calls

➤ *Your friend is a distributor for a supplement you believe is of high quality and is said to boost energy and help certain physical problems. You have taken these vitamins and feel very enthusiastic about their value. Your friend encourages you to become a distributor and sell them to your clients.*

Is it ethical to sell products to a client? Some practitioners have no qualms about selling vitamins, blue-green algae, or magnets to clients. Others don't think it's a good idea. How do you decide what is right? And what do you do if your employer encourages or requires you to try to sell products to clients? I've heard stories of employers that have quotas for the staff to meet, at peril of losing their job if they can't (or won't) sell.

Bear in mind that nutritional counseling is not within the scope of practice of massage therapy. Selling *anything* usually involves some level of explanation to the client. Telling someone "Take two every morning and two every evening," is prescribing—even if it's a nonprescription drug. As massage therapists, we are not allowed to tell people to take an over-the-counter aspirin for their aches and pains, so how are we allowed to tell them to take a vitamin? What's the difference? Anyone can walk into a store and buy an aspirin or buy vitamins without any prescription or advice about using it, and that's where we stand to get in trouble—giving that advice.

Looking back at the list of questions that you want to keep in mind, you can probably see a number of potential problems with selling goods to clients. The main ethical issue isn't whether it may benefit the client to use the product that you sell; it's whether you are unfairly using the power of the therapeutic relationship. Is the client really free to refuse, or would they make a purchase mainly to please you? Aside from the ethical considerations, even subtly attempting to sell products to clients could make some clients feel pressured and uncomfortable.

Another issue is that selling anything to a client other than the professional services you have contracted for creates a dual relationship, which complicates the interaction between you and the client. Suppose a client to whom you have sold vitamins doesn't benefit as much as you led her to expect. That could damage your working relationship. If your employer wants you to push clients to buy products, you might try getting them to change their policy by arguing that a hard sell will surely offend many clients. Working for someone who has different professional standards puts you in a bind between your obligation to your employer and your wish to be a conscientious professional. As noted before, it's wise to check out such policies before you agree to a job.

Ethical Retailing

Although any retailing automatically places you in a dual relationship with clients, there are some parameters that you can adhere to that will eliminate potential problems, if you're the business owner and have control over the situation.

REAL EXPERIENCE

I was working in a busy day spa. Although it was not the case when I was hired, the owner got involved in a multilevel marketing company about a year after I came to work there, and put in a big display of their products in the lobby. He expected all the therapists to push the products, which ran the gamut from essential oils, skin and hair care, nutritional supplements, and weight loss products. It was my opinion that it was all expensive and overpriced. When he first got involved with the company, he held a staff meeting and told the other massage therapists and me that we were all expected to sell, sell, sell. He insisted that we use essential oils for every massage. He said we should convince every client that they needed to be taking the supplements for their health. If anyone was overweight, even by 10 pounds (and whose call is that?), we were supposed to be selling them the weight loss products. He had scripts for us to memorize so we would know exactly what to say when trying to make a sale. He basically expected us to turn the whole appointment into a sales pitch. I hated it, and so did everyone else who worked there.

When I came to work there, there were security cameras at the front and rear entrances, and one at the front desk where people checked in and out. The final straw for me happened one day just after closing time. All the clients had gone and the therapists were getting ready to leave when he called everyone out to the front desk. He put the security video on the computer screen and turned it around so everyone could see it, and proceeded to go on a rant. The screen showed me walking toward the front desk with a client, thanking her for coming, and telling her that the receptionist would set her up with a future appointment. "Just look at yourself, Robert! This woman is FAT and you didn't even attempt to sell her the weight loss shakes! You need to start doing a lot better!" I just snapped. I told him that I was a massage therapist, not a snake oil salesman, and I quit. Another therapist said she was quitting, too, and we both went out the door, leaving the owner standing there with his mouth open. The other therapist and I ended up renting space together and opening our own business—where we don't sell anything at all. It's a lot less stressful and we both enjoy going to work now.

—R.J., LMT

- Avoid discussing products in the treatment room unless in response to a direct question from a client, such as "Do you offer these neck pillows for sale?" Answer but don't go into a sales pitch. A simple "Yes, and I'll be glad to show them to you before you leave," is sufficient. If a client *asks* you for a product you used with them during treatment, and you don't retail, it's perfectly fine to tell them where to obtain it, or offer to order it for them.

- Never tell a client that they *need* anything you are selling.
- Avoid retailing any product that makes health or beauty claims—and avoid making any yourself. Weight loss products, products that claim to remove wrinkles, or get rid of cellulite or other such claims are a problem waiting to happen. A product that claims to moisturize the skin and one that claims to make you look 20 years younger are two different things.

Refusing to Work with a Client or Stopping Work with a Client

The Ethical Standard

Practitioners in private practice have a right of refusal. They can refuse to work with a prospective client or to discontinue working with a client if they think that they cannot form a therapeutic alliance with that client or if they do not have the training or physical capabilities to work with that client. If you are not self-employed, your employer may not think you have that right—yet another reason to choose your employer carefully.

Judgment Calls

➤ *Your regular client arrives, having spent the afternoon doing yard work, and is uncharacteristically dirty and sweaty.*

➤ *You have worked with a couple on outcall basis several times. While you are alone with the husband, he makes suggestive remarks.*

➤ *You weigh 100 pounds. Your prospective client weighs twice that and has requested deep work. You don't think that you can give the depth of massage that he wants.*

There are many reasons (outside contraindications, of course) you may choose not to work with a client. Poor hygiene, inappropriate sexual behavior, or a physical mismatch for you are three reasons. (Granted that a small massage therapist can, with good body mechanics, handle deep work with any size client; however, it's up to each therapist to decide his or her physical boundaries.) There are other reasons clients may not be appropriate for your work or may be beyond your abilities. They may be mentally ill or may have physical conditions that make the kind of work you do unsuitable for them. You want to be aware of what those conditions are and of what your own physical and emotional limitations are. In addition to not taking

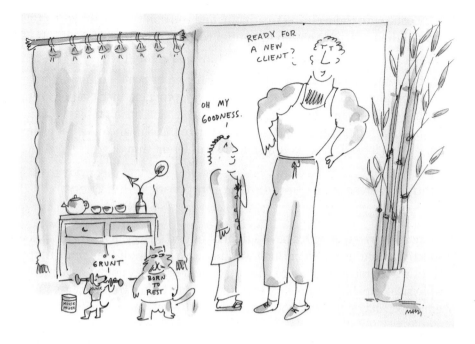

on clients with conditions that aren't appropriate for your kind of work, you also may want to limit the number of clients you see who present special difficulties, whether emotional or physical. These include clients who need extra help or reassurance and who take extra time in terms of phone calls and consultations outside their sessions or clients who are in acute physical distress.

Regarding the situation with the sweaty client, most practitioners probably wouldn't mind working with an occasionally grimy client. Those who do mind need to make their policies clear up front to avoid the embarrassment of turning away a client. Spelling out these policies on an intake application form is a good way to get the point across. For instance, some massage therapy clinics post a notice or have clients sign a statement that says the therapists can refuse to work with someone or can terminate work because of a client's poor hygiene or inappropriate sexual behavior or comments.

In the case of the husband who made inappropriate remarks, it depends on your prior relationship with that person and the degree of offensiveness of the remarks. If, for instance, a client makes obvious offensive or degrading remarks, you should stop working with him at once—both stop the session and decline to make another appointment. If you are not clear about the person's intent or think he may just be testing you, you can give him a warning that you will not continue working with him unless he stops being suggestive. (Exceptions can be made for a regular client who makes a sexually oriented joke that's clearly not meant to be disrespectful and that doesn't offend you.) In this case, if the husband had never been inappropriate before, you could say, "I don't work with clients who don't treat me with respect. I'll end the massage if you make any more remarks like that." If he continues, you need to end the massage and let him know you won't work with him again. You might lose the wife's business also, but there's never a good reason to work with a disrespectful client. When you decide not to take on someone who you think taxes your physical capabilities, you can be straightforward about your reasons: "I can't do justice to someone your size. May I give you the names of some practitioners who would be more appropriate?"

Sometimes you may not want to work with clients because they have emotional needs that you are not trained to handle—perhaps they are deeply depressed or working with issues of childhood abuse. Even if clients are working with a psychotherapist, you may still feel you would not be suited to work with them; for instance, you may feel overwhelmed about working with someone who frequently cries. It takes sensitivity to refer such clients to another massage therapist without them feeling rejected (see "Clients Who Are Emotional or Want Advice" in Chapter 6).

Confidentiality

The Ethical Standard

Nothing a client says or does—and no information we have about a client—should be revealed to others without the client's permission unless disclosure is required by law or court order or is necessary for the protection of the public. Situations in which we can—and, in fact, are often obligated to—legally breach confidentiality are those in which there is clear and imminent danger to the client or others, there is suspicion of abuse or neglect of a child or incapacitated person, or there is a medical emergency.

Judgment Calls

Specific procedures for keeping patient information private are discussed in Chapter 3. However, there are some common ways that practitioners can violate confidentiality if they don't understand the finer points.

For instance, in the situation discussed earlier in which the husband made sexually inappropriate remarks, what do you say to his wife if you decide not to continue to work with the husband? She's also your client, and you've been scheduling their appointments back-to-back at their home. The standards of confidentiality dictate that if the wife asks why you stopped seeing her husband, you can't tell her the reason. You can't even imply or suggest it. You can't tell her that her husband is an unfaithful womanizer. You have to say, "Even though he is your husband, I can't ethically talk about another client." If you've told her about your standards at the outset, it makes reinforcing the policy easier. The chances are pretty good she's going to figure it out—her version of it, anyway. She may conclude that her husband came on to you. Or she may conclude that you came on to him! Either way, it's an awkward situation, and you may need to dismiss both of them as clients, especially if you are going to encounter him during future visits to their home. Violations of confidentiality can happen quickly. Here's an example: Mary and Susie are friends, and both are clients of Joe, a massage therapist. Mary says to Joe, "I haven't seen Susie in a while. How's she doing?" It's easy for Joe to say, "Oh, she's still having a hard time with her husband. She had to get a restraining order against him." But if he does, he's broken confidentiality with Susie. To make it worse, now Mary knows that Joe passes on clients' private information to other people. Even "Susie's feeling great" is a violation. To keep clear framework, Joe can say lightly, "Oh, you know I can't talk about my other clients." Clients who are friends with other clients may sometimes test you—usually not consciously—to see if you will talk about their friend to them (and, therefore, talk to the friend about them).

Here's another way that practitioners can easily violate confidentiality. Quite often, if one client has referred a friend who then also becomes a client, the practitioner thanks the referrer, thereby letting them know that their friend is now a client. Although this is a common practice and it seems both harmless and good business manners to express gratitude, you might want to rethink it. Doesn't it violate the new client's privacy? If a client says, "I told Dave about you. Did he ever call?" You want to thank the client for making the referral, but you shouldn't reveal whether Dave called or not. Just because the client made a referral, Dave's interactions with you don't become his business. You can say, "I appreciate your referral, and I understand why you want to know if he followed up. However, all my interactions with clients are confidential, so I can't tell you whether Dave called or not." When you first talk with a prospective client who has been referred by a friend or another client, you can ask permission to thank the friend for the referral. Some massage therapists may have the question on their intake form, "Is there someone we can thank for referring you to us?" If they give permission, it's fine to thank the referring friend, but you should still refrain from sharing anything else about them or their sessions with you.

Clients may want to keep private the fact that they are seeing a manual therapist for all kinds of reasons, such as not wanting to let their spouse know how they are spending money or fearing that someone else might think having a massage is a shady or self-indulgent practice.

If you see clients (past or present) in an outside setting, standard protocol is to not be the first to approach. Some clients may not have told their friends or family that they are seeing a massage therapist, and they may not want to have to explain to their companion who you are. If they acknowledge you, then you can match their level of friendliness. For instance, if a client merely nods to you, you can nod back but don't engage them in conversation. Even if the client is alone, they may not want to have their privacy invaded.

Sometimes you may be tempted to name-drop when a well-known or famous person is or has been a client. Famous people appreciate their privacy and have a right to it. Name-dropping is rarely impressive and only reveals the practitioner as someone who does not safeguard clients' privacy.

There's another aspect of confidentiality that relates to your own self-care. Clients sometimes share things we wish we they hadn't. We hear about their cancer diagnoses, the loss of a family member or the burden of taking care of one, the problems with their spouse and their children, as well as with their money, their in-laws, their job, and the list just goes on. In between that, and our genuine sympathy for people who are in pain, whether physically, emotionally, or both, is the need to keep ourselves from emotional overload. We can do that by taking care of ourselves, making time to enjoy our hobbies and our recreation, not overworking ourselves, and seeking supervision from a mentor when we need it. Getting ongoing bodywork for yourself also helps with emotional overload.

However, talking with friends or colleagues about clients as a way of venting isn't a good idea. The possibility of giving away information or identifying a client by accident is too great. Especially in a rural area or small community, the therapist may know who you are talking about even if you don't mention their name.

It may be difficult to be strict about confidentiality if you are not self-employed. In a spa or even a physician's or chiropractor's office, policies about when it's OK to share information about clients can be unclear or careless. In a spa, both staff and massage therapists may see nothing wrong with gossiping about clients; therapists may readily disclose information they learned during a private session. Your choice, then, is to participate or not, keeping in mind how you would feel if you were the client. It may seem sometimes like harmless venting about a difficult client, but it's disrespectful of both the client and professional standards.

Sharing information relevant to the work is a different matter. It's useful to the client if therapists share, either verbally or in chart notes, what kind of massage a client prefers, for instance. The management still needs to get permission from clients for any information being revealed about them between therapists.

CONSIDER THIS

A massage therapist found out that the receptionist where he worked was saying derogatory things about clients on Facebook, and even though she wasn't naming names, she would describe them in unflattering terms like this "You should have seen this woman that came in today! 300 pounds at least...she looked like a stuffed sausage in those purple pants she was wearing!" When the therapist said she needed to stop it, she said "I'm not a massage therapist. I'm not worried about confidentiality!" When he complained to the owner, he was told to just mind his own business. What would you have done? Nothing? Call the clients and tell them? Look for another job?

Other Ethical Standards and Implementation

Some ethics guidelines are fairly straightforward; we just need help with implementing them.

False Claims

The Ethical Standard

Making false claims or inflated promises is unethical. It is unethical to obtain clients by persuasion or influence or to use comments about our services that contain untrue statements. It is unethical to create inflated or unjustified expectations of favorable results.

Implementation

In describing your work to prospective clients, be honest about your work's limits and about any possible negative side effects. Never guarantee results. You can speak of the benefits that you know to be true. For instance, you could say (assuming that it is true to the best of your knowledge) that "many people" have felt calmer, more flexible, more energetic, and so forth after having a massage or a certain kind of bodywork. You can state that "many people" have experienced alleviation of general symptoms. But be aware of the dangers of even subtly leading clients to expect specific cures or fixes. The causes of physical problems are complex, and the outcome of treatments can't be predicted. A colleague says:

➤ *Any time I've done an oversell about the benefits of my method of bodywork, it comes back to haunt me. My reasons are usually well-intentioned. Sometimes I'm tempted to do a "hard sell" because I really like a prospective client and want to be able to help him. I believe strongly in my work, and sometimes that makes me promise too much. I think it always backfires on me. That will be the client who doesn't get any relief from the treatment.*

Scope of Practice

The Ethical Standard

Exceeding our **scope of practice** is unethical and often dangerous to our clients. It is unethical to represent ourselves as having training or expertise that we do not possess, such as suggesting that we are skilled in handling serious medical conditions.

Scope of practice:
The traditional knowledge base and standard practices of the profession.

We have an obligation to refer clients to appropriately trained professionals and, with the client's permission, to consult with other professionals who are treating our clients. If we have a client who is ill and currently receiving medical treatment for a serious problem, we should consult with the client's primary practitioner (with the client's permission) before beginning working.

Implementation

Practitioners who exceed the scope of their practice are a cause of concern for their colleagues because they reflect poorly on the profession. Some bodyworkers claim to work with emotional and psychological issues, but they have had no training or supervision in these areas. Some bodyworkers claim to have the skills to perform a complex manual technique with only limited training in it. One weekend workshop (or even a few) doesn't make one an expert in anything. It's unethical to advertise ourselves, either on our business cards or verbally, as proficient in a method for which we have only a superficial knowledge or training.

We need to respect the time and training it takes to become a psychotherapist, osteopath, medical doctor, chiropractor, physical therapist, and so forth. At the same time, we need to respect the value of our own skills. Practitioners of other disciplines often have many more years of training than we do—in their discipline. Other health-care practitioners may be allowed to diagnose, and prescribe, and perform surgery—things that we're not able to do. But we have a skill that they are lacking—and we need to stick to it. Giving people advice we are not qualified to give is a gross violation of the scope of practice. Another of our unique gifts as health-care professionals is the amount of time we spend with our clients and the level of attention and care we give them. There is plenty of healing in simply being with people in a conscious, attentive way—listening to them, listening to their bodies. If we appreciate the strength and value of our own work, we won't feel the need to pad our resumes

If we appreciate the strength and value of our own work, we won't feel the need to pad our resumes.

Informed Consent

The Ethical Standard

We need to have clients' **informed consent** for (1) the basic treatment or kind of manual therapy that we offer, (2) any work that is near clients' genitals or anus or a woman's breasts, (3) any work that is near an area that we know to be sensitive or triggering for a particular client, and (4) anything we do that is different from the work we have contracted to do or that the client expects from us.

Informed consent:
A client's authorization for services to be performed by a practitioner. The client or the client's guardian must be fully advised of what the service will entail and its benefits and contraindications, and he or she must be competent to give consent.

This means that clients are aware of both the possible benefits and the possible side effects of our work. For instance, they may need to be told that when the body is healing naturally, sometimes they feel worse before they feel better. Clients also need to know the reasons for a specific treatment or why we need to work in a sensitive area. They also need to be capable of understanding our explanations at the time—they cannot be deeply in an altered state, for instance.

Implementation

Some practitioners obtain written consent (and some states may require that consent be written) from new clients before they begin work. They use a form that explains what the general benefits of the work are, assures clients that there are no guarantees, and states that no medical treatment or diagnosis is involved. Having a client sign such a form also is excellent protection for practitioners. Although it isn't a legal document, it can be a deterrent to lawsuits.

In an intake interview, clients should also be told, either in writing or verbally, about any contraindications to the type of work you do. As you are working, explain and get agreement for any work that is potentially unsettling, such as work near the genitals. If you decide to use a different method than what has been agreed on, explain the method and get the client's consent. It is always the client's choice, and that must be respected. Giving a deep massage to someone who requested light work, or doing energy work that the client doesn't want just because you want to do it, is not being client centered—and we should always be client centered.

A key to the idea of consent is the understanding that because of transference, clients are not as free to say no as they would ordinarily be. This is especially true if they are already on the table. For this reason, it's best to get clients' consent for new methods *before* sessions begin and to be clear with clients that they can ask you to stop or can refuse a treatment at any time. If you have an urge to try something different after the session is under way, find a way to ask permission that isn't disruptive and that as much as possible allows the client to refuse.

A friend relates:

➤ *In the middle of a session with a massage therapist I had seen before, I was jolted out of my relaxed state by a noisy and teeth-rattling large electric massager on my back. The massage therapist had never used it before, so it was an unpleasant surprise. I suffered in silence for a while and finally asked him to please stop. He said, "Oh, sorry, I couldn't remember if I'd used this on you before." I didn't say anything, but I was thinking, "So, why didn't you ask me?" That therapist could have said, "Some clients like for me to use an electric percussive massager on their backs because of the strength of it. Others find it to be too much. It's fine with me if you don't want me to use it. Would you like to try it?" (And the massage therapist could have noted in the client's records whether electric massagers were part of her treatment.)*

We need to obtain permission from clients for any addition we make that may be unexpected or unfamiliar. Here are a few complaints from clients:

➤ *Before he began working, my massage therapist began chanting. I didn't understand what he was doing. Although it freaked me out, I didn't say anything.*

➤ *My massage therapist held her hands over my body for several minutes without doing anything. I had come for a relaxing massage and felt like she was wasting my time and money.*

➤ *My therapist started laying a line of crystals up the center of my body as soon as she came into the room. I asked her what she was doing and she claimed she was balancing my chakras. I didn't even know I had chakras.*

In the above-mentioned cases, the massage therapists could have avoided problems if they had asked the client's permission to add their own personal rituals to the massage. That includes saying (out loud) any kind of prayer, which may be offensive to some. If you have such a ritual, explain what you want to do in simple, nonmystic terms, letting the client know how long it will take and assuring them that it won't cut into their massage session time—and it shouldn't. A client who has booked an hour of massage should have the expectation of getting an hour of massage—not 45 minutes of massage and 15 minutes of your personal rituals or energy work that they haven't asked for, just because that's what *you* want to do. Asking them after they're already on the table is placing the client in the position where they are already undressed, already in a vulnerable position, viewing you as the authority figure, and taking advantage of the power differential. Discuss it before taking them to the treatment room.

For instance, you could say, "I find that a few minutes of doing deep breathing exercises can help me get centered before a massage. It'll only take a few minutes but if it makes you at all uncomfortable, I don't need to do it. Of course, you won't be charged for the extra time." Or "Sometimes I like to incorporate energy work into my massage. It may not look or feel like I'm doing anything other than holding my hands over your body, but the few minutes it takes won't take away from your massage time. Do I have your permission to try that or would you rather I just stick with the regular massage? It's up to you." Repeat: the client is paying for this time, and it is *their* time.

Straddling the categories of both the need for informed consent and staying within our scope of practice is the all-too-common practice of telling clients our intuitive or "psychic" notions about them. Unless you advertise yourself as a psychic offering such services to clients, you want to avoid telling a client who has come for a comforting massage (or any other kind of bodywork) that, for instance, she holds anger in her belly. (Maybe a client would welcome hearing our intuitive sense that she holds cheerfulness in her belly, but for some reason, all too often such psychic pronouncements about clients are negative and unflattering, and they also verge on the out-of-scope practice of psychology.) Remember that clients usually won't tell us when we make them uncomfortable, so it's up to us to be sure to obtain their permission before making unexpected or intrusive additions to the session. Otherwise, they may express their discomfort by just declining to make another appointment with you, and seeking someone who won't impose their own belief systems and wishes onto them.

Disrespect of Other Professionals

The Ethical Standard

It's unethical to imply that our skill level or our method of manual therapy is superior to either another practitioner's or another kind of bodywork.

Implementation

If you malign another practitioner, it could make you look insecure in your client's eyes. Also, if you make critical remarks about a practitioner your client is seeing or has seen, you are questioning not only that practitioner's competence, but also the client's judgment. You want to avoid careless talk, gossip, personal remarks, and assessments about the skills of another practitioner. We all have ex-clients who think we're skilled and compassionate and those who do not. Take care with another practitioner's reputation

We all have ex-clients who think we're skilled and compassionate and those who do not. Take care with another practitioner's reputation.

The same goes for maligning other kinds of manual therapies or alternative health practices or being disrespectful of the medical profession. Doing so would make you look small and could offend clients who are loyal to that kind of treatment. If a client *asks you* what you think of a modality that you believe is sheer bunk, you can answer honestly without going on a diatribe about it, such as "I don't personally believe in the principles of _____, but many people do."

Going on a rant about the medical profession to a client is not only unprofessional, but could be dangerous to the client as well. Persuading someone that they shouldn't get their child vaccinated because you personally choose that path is wrong. Telling someone that they should refuse to take the treatment or the medication a doctor has prescribed for them is wrong. You are not a doctor. You do not know more than a doctor. Acting as an authority on medicine is beyond scope of practice and unethical, regardless of your personal beliefs. If the word gets around about that, you may find that not only have you killed any chances of getting referrals from doctors, you may also find yourself brought before the board for practicing medicine without a license—or worse. A naturopath in the town next to mine advised parents to stop giving their diabetic child insulin and follow his protocol instead. The child died, and the naturopath went to prison.

If a client speaks negatively about another practitioner, you need to stay objective. Either remain silent or make a comment related to the client's feelings, such as, "It sounds as if it was an uncomfortable experience for you." You might also ask the clients if they think their feelings about the previous practitioner could interfere with their ability to enjoy your work. If so, you can suggest that they find a way to get closure with the other practitioner. You can say, "I can't comment about another practitioner's work, but I see that you are still upset and it might be useful to both you and the practitioner if you would write or call him and let him know why you were dissatisfied."

Staying Out of Trouble

Lawsuits And Ethics Complaints

Ethics and the perception of what is ethical are not determined by impersonal rules. They are grounded in your relationship with your clients. In general, if you violate a rule of ethics, you cross a boundary—you go outside the safety of the professional relationship. The more you stay inside professional framework and boundaries and the more you honor the therapeutic relationship, the less likely you are to get into serious trouble.

The more you stay inside professional framework and boundaries and the more you honor the therapeutic relationship, the less likely you are to get into serious trouble.

Lawsuits, Ethics Complaints, and the Therapeutic Relationship

Many ethics complaints and lawsuits against practitioners have little to do with the practitioners' technical skills and a good deal to do with whether the practitioners appear to care about their clients.

A study published in a medical journal showed that a doctor was more likely to be sued if patients felt the doctor was rushing visits, not answering questions, or being rude in some other way. A comparison between doctors who had been sued and those who had not showed no difference in the level of competence of the two groups as perceived by their colleagues. However, the ones who had never been sued were more likely to be seen by their patients as concerned, accessible, and willing to communicate (Hickson GB, Federspiel CF, Pichert JW, et al. Patient complaints and malpractice risk. *J Am Med Assoc.* 2002;287:3003–3005).

Practitioners need to respond in a professional, caring manner to clients who have complaints. Sometimes practitioners make the mistake of stonewalling these clients—not returning their calls or refusing to talk with them. Failing to respond to disappointed or angry clients usually makes things worse. Aside from being an unethical way to handle clients' grievances, this type of behavior usually makes clients angrier, sometimes to the point of filing an ethics complaint. Also, if you do not listen to clients with grievances, you deny yourself the opportunity to learn from their feedback.

While you may not subscribe to the old adage, "The customer is always right," the best thing you can do is *listen* to their complaint. People will sometimes forgive a lapse in judgment or behavior, or a perceived fault, from a practitioner, or when the practitioner at least gives them the opportunity to speak to them about it. They will usually not forgive someone who ignores them altogether.

An administrator for a bodywork school who handles complaints against its graduates agrees that practitioners need to be accessible and open. She says that quite often bodyworkers could avoid having complaints lodged against them if they would simply answer clients' phone calls and allow grievances to be aired. Clients have to be upset or angry in order to file a complaint. In many cases, practitioners who are complained against have followed normal ethical standards but have angered clients by seeming indifferent to their feelings or by emotionally abandoning them in some way. Unless clients are abusive or harassing, the best thing you can do, even if you feel you committed no error, is to allow them to speak their minds and let them know that you regret their dissatisfaction.

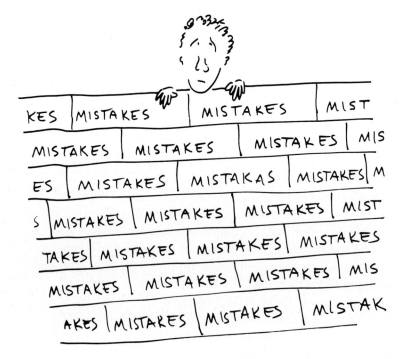

Framework Exceptions: A Red Flag

Practitioners who have made mistakes or have been complained against have usually had a pattern of making small boundary errors in general or have been careless about boundaries with one particular client. It should be a red flag for you when you're tempted to go outside your own standard policies or the standard practices in your community.

When There Are No Warning Signs: The Need for Documentation and Professional Association

There are instances of practitioners being sued or complained against when there were no significant warning signs. (Individual circumstances of ethics complaints vary. Practitioners who have been officially complained against or threatened with a lawsuit should consult an attorney and work with the ethics boards of their organizations.) Two things saved them in court: they had carefully documented the client's presenting problems and course of treatment, and they had the backing of a professional association. You need to keep careful notes, especially when you feel uneasy about a client, when you work with clients with medical issues, and when you work with clients who have been abused. But since you never know which client may end up unhappy with your services, it makes sense to keep careful records on all clients, and in regulated states, keeping records is the law. The importance of documentation cannot be stressed enough.

REAL EXPERIENCE

A new client wanted me to give her a discount simply because she said she couldn't afford my prices, although she was working and appeared to be driving a new car. I don't usually give discounts except to those who are disabled, so I refused her at first but eventually gave in because she was so insistent. What a mistake! She turned out to be constantly demanding and complaining, and I never felt that she was satisfied with the work. Although I offered to refer her to another practitioner, she stayed with me through several sessions, complaining all the while. After she stopped coming to me, she filed a complaint with my professional association, saying that my work wasn't useful to her and that I had knowingly cheated her. I found out too late that she had had this same pattern with other practitioners in the area. I learned the lesson that bending my own boundaries and policies for people usually turns out worse than if I had been firm about not making exceptions just because a client keeps whining or demanding that I do so.

—Anonymous MT

Belonging to a professional association (which generally means they may also be providing you with liability insurance as part of your member benefits) is also helpful. Clients' attorneys will want to make a manual therapy practitioner look sinister, dishonest, or fly-by-night. Belonging to a respected national group enhances practitioners' image. In addition, professional associations often provide witnesses to back up the legitimacy of our methods.

The professional associations usually do not, however, come to the defense of massage therapists accused of sexual impropriety with a client.

The Right Thing

What's right may vary depending on the client and the situation. How strictly do we interpret the guideline, for instance, that it's not ethical to benefit personally from a client? No one is going to haul us into court if we have cleverly placed our dying ficus plant in the middle of the room, hoping our next client, a regular of many years and the owner of a plant shop, will notice it and give us good advice. If the plant shop owner was a new client and we met him at the door with a barrage of questions about our ailing flora, again, we probably wouldn't be sued, but we might lose him as a client or at least make him uneasy.

However, if we use our influence with a regular client to get him to invest in our plant business, we could end up in court with that client if the business fails (or even if it doesn't). To stay out of trouble and avoid taking advantage of our clients, we need a solid understanding of relationship dynamics and the rules of ethics that our profession asks us to follow.

Manual therapies are becoming increasingly popular, and respect for the profession is growing along with its popularity. Each new phase of our professional growth gives us opportunities to use our new power and strength in ways that will benefit our clients and enhance the image of the profession.

Questions for Reflection

1. Everyone has some kind of prejudice; your goal is to be aware of what yours are. Think about the ways that you prejudge people based on their appearance, skin color, clothes, or what you think their beliefs to be. Are any of your judgments so severe that you would not want to work with a particular group of people? What can you do to become more understanding of that group, or do you stubbornly refuse to even consider their point of view?

2. Has a professional ever violated your confidentiality in a small way, for instance, by letting someone else know that you are his or her client or that you enjoyed a session? How did that feel to you? Has a professional ever told you something about a client that violated the client's confidentiality? Did that influence the way you felt about the practitioner's professionalism? In what way?

3. Have you ever used the services of a professional (massage therapist, bodyworker, chiropractor, physician, or so forth) or any kind of service person (plumber or carpenter) who claimed to know more than he or she really did or who claimed to be able to help you in ways that he or she couldn't? What did you learn from that experience?

4. Have you ever been to a professional who bad-mouthed another professional or said that his or her own work was superior to that of another professional? What did you learn from that experience?

thePoint To learn more about the concepts discussed in this chapter, visit http://thePoint.lww.com/Allen-McIntosh4e

CHAPTER 6

Boundaries and the Power of Words

We communicate with clients in more than words; everything we do speaks volumes to our clients about our professional attitudes and values. Clean, warm offices and a welcoming smile say one thing, and their absence says another. The way we touch can communicate "I'm so interested in working with you and helping you" or "Here's just another bunch of tight muscles."

There is a constant conversation between practitioner and client—much of it nonverbal—about the basic questions of intention and role: "What are the two of us doing in this room together?" This chapter is about the verbal side of that conversation: what we say to clients and how we understand what are they saying to us.

The Power of Our Words

Two powerful influences give our words to clients more weight than they would ordinarily have:

- Transference: As explained in Chapter 4, there is an inherent power differential in the therapeutic relationship, and clients are likely to unconsciously relate to us as an authority or a parent figure.

- **Altered state**: During sessions, clients are more open than usual, less defended, and closer to their unconscious minds; our words can sink in more deeply.

Altered state:
A state of consciousness in which we are more deeply relaxed, less aware of our thinking minds, and more open and vulnerable than we are in our day-to-day functioning.

Because of these two influences, clients may have a heightened sensitivity to what we say. Whether we're in private practice or work for someone else, clients may be more affected by our words than they ordinarily would be. They may, for instance, hear us as being critical when that is not our intention. Our words can be deflating to a client if they sound negative or judgmental.

Here's an example of a client's reaction:

➤ *I'm never going back to that massage therapist. He made me feel fat and un-attractive. While he was working near my stomach, he said, "I'm sure you're aware of the unhealthy effects of being overweight."*
Compassionate words can have an equally strong effect:

➤ *When my bodyworker said, "I know you've had a rough week. I hope I can be helpful to you," I felt myself relax before she even touched me.*

Our words can touch clients' hearts or sink their spirits.

Our words can touch clients' hearts or sink their spirits.

Attitudes and Roles

This chapter gives suggestions for useful phrases for common problematic situations with clients. Although we can learn some words to say, no one can hand us a surefire script that will guarantee good results. The words we choose reflect our attitudes about both our clients and our roles. If we understand our roles, the right attitude and the right words will follow.

➤ *A client shows up 15 minutes late. One practitioner says, "You're always late. My time is just as valuable as yours. I wish you would start coming on time."*

➤ *Another says, "We only have 45 minutes left in your hour, but I can help you get rid of lots of stress during that time."*

We can hear the difference in their attitudes and in their ideas about their roles. The second practitioner sounds like a professional talking with another adult who needs both education and nurturing. They manage to do two important things at once: set appropriate limits with the underlying message, "You don't get a full hour if you show up late," while showing concern for the client with the underlying message, "I want to help you feel better." They take care of their professional needs by not letting the client take advantage of them while they also take care of the client's legitimate needs for help.

The first practitioner starts out sounding like a martyred parent scolding a bad child and then ends up sounding like a whiny child herself. The practitioner's statements focus on their own discomfort. They also sound caught up in countertransference: that is, they seem to be taking the client's lateness personally and forgetting their professional role. Since the clearer we are about our role, the less likely we are to react in a personal way, we need to take another look at our professional role in light of communications.

Boundary Lessons

A client who was late for her very first appointment didn't seem to be upset about it when I said we only had 45 minutes left to do the intake and her massage. However, when she was checking out and making another appointment, she said "I'd like to get the last appointment of the day. That way, it won't matter if I'm late." I immediately said "Ma'am, I make it a point to be at home by 6 p.m. in order to have dinner with my family. If you are late for the last appointment of the day, you will still only receive the time that is left on your hour, and the charge is for the full hour." She looked incredulous and said "My old massage therapist was a lot more accommodating!" I stood my ground and told her I hoped she could understand that my policies are what they are, and that if she couldn't accept them, she'd be happier going elsewhere. She immediately told me I had given a great massage and she would go ahead and make the appointment. She has been coming for a year now and has been on time most of that time, but I know if I had caved in and ignored her being late, she would have taken full advantage of it.

—A.E., LMT

The Professional Role: Dictator versus Compassionate Practitioner

To better understand our role, we need to return to the basics of the therapeutic relationship: the concepts of paying attention to the contract, being client centered, being responsible for a safe environment, and maintaining our own rights. If we don't keep those in mind, we may end up sounding more like little dictators than compassionate professionals—or alternatively, find ourselves in the position of letting people take advantage of us, and becoming resentful of our work.

A common mistake for practitioners (like the first practitioner above) is inadvertently treating clients as if they were wayward children who need to be controlled and ordered around rather than as adults who have come for our professional care and concern. (Clients do need clear structure and information, but we can provide those things in a respectful way.) Here are some examples of the "little dictator" attitude:

➤ *Bodyworker Barbara relates, "I'm disgusted with my out-of-shape client who won't do any of the exercises I've given him. I need to tell him that just getting a massage won't help him much if he won't follow up at home."*

Aside from being dismayed by Barbara's negative judgment about her client, our concern is whether Barbara has an agreement with the client to assign him

---

REAL EXPERIENCE

A man and his wife were both clients. They were in their early 60s; both still worked and were active people. Although they were both slightly over-weight, maybe by 15 to 20 pounds, they otherwise appeared healthy. Ac-cording to their intake forms and interviews, neither was on any medication. One day as the man was checking out after his appointment, he said, "I really wish you would talk to my wife about her weight. She has put some on in the past few years." He was totally oblivious to the fact that *he* was carrying as many extra pounds as his wife! I just looked at him and politely said "I'm afraid I'll have to decline. That's not my area of expertise or in my scope of practice to advise people about their weight. Maybe you could suggest she gets a checkup." It's not my place to do that, and I was nice about it, but I let him know it.

—K.B., CMT

---

exercises—and whether that's even within her scope of practice. You may *suggest* that stretching, walking, or whatever may help the client, but *you don't have the right to assign them anything.* That crosses the line into prescribing. If the client does not want any service other than a massage, then Barbara is doubly out of bounds, first by deciding what is "best" for him and then by being annoyed when he doesn't do what she thinks he should.

If a practitioner believes that he or she has other services or expertise that would be helpful to the client, he or she can say, preferably during the initial intake, "You're already helping your health a great deal by coming to get a massage. Just to let you know what else is available, I also offer my services as a personal trainer (or whatever service) if you are interested."

Since saying even that little might come across as a negative judgment to an out-of-shape client, a better alternative may be to educate clients by spelling out our services in a brochure that we give to clients or by directing clients to our web-site, if we have one.

➤ *Somatic practitioner Sam says, "My client has such a control problem. She wants to tell me how to do the music, the lighting, even where I can touch her. I tell her that I can't do my best if she won't let me work the way I want to."*

Who really has the control problem here? Sam has forgotten that he is respon-sible for creating an emotionally and physically safe and comfortable environment for the client and that the client's needs are paramount. Certainly, this client has a right to her preferences about music and lighting, within reason, and she has a right to say that she would prefer that the bodyworker not work with some areas of her body. He's making the session all about him, when it's supposed to be all about the client.

Suppose a client had a request for where we should or shouldn't work and we think that honoring that request wouldn't serve her well. For instance, her shoulders and neck are hurting, and she wants us to focus most of the session there. We would then need to try to educate her: "Although you feel your tension in your shoulders and neck, they are part of a larger tension pattern. It would probably be more effective for your shoulders and neck pain if we take a whole-body approach."

Of course, if a client wants us not to work on a certain area for reasons of modesty or privacy, we are obligated to honor that request. We may not fully understand the reasons for a client's sensitivities, but we are obliged to comply cheerfully and without taking personal offense.

Communicating with Clients

In light of the basics of the professional relationship, here are general guidelines and suggestions for talking with clients. Of course, you want to find your own style and words.

CONSIDER THIS

Have you ever had an experience with a massage therapist who didn't listen? I have. I once went to a massage therapist with the complaint that my neck was stiff and sore. She worked me over good—everywhere except where I had told her I was hurting! As the hour dwindled away I kept wondering when she was going to work on my neck, and I finally asked her. She said "You had more serious problems elsewhere. We'll have to get to it next time." I was so upset when I left, and of course I never went back. The next day I called another therapist, told her about the experience, and that I needed neck work. She ended up being my therapist for the next few years until she moved. The first therapist closed her business a year or two after I visited her. Even though we need to work with the related muscles, and not just spend the whole hour where the pain might be, we need to keep in mind that most clients are not anatomy experts, and we may need to explain to them why we're working in other areas first, and we definitely need to pay attention to the area they said was hurting. When we don't listen to clients, or when they feel we aren't listening to them due to our own lack of clear communication about what we're doing, we make a very bad impression.

Use the Client's Words

When you ask clients during your intake procedure what they want to get from the massage, note how they talk about their bodies, their discomfort, or their lives. Using their own words and images when talking with them will have more impact than using yours. This is a simple but very effective way to quickly establish a connection with clients and to let them know you are listening to them and value their input. For example, "I understand your neck is hurting, and particularly bothers you when you've been at the computer all day, is that right?"

Talk in Terms of What the Client's Values Are

Clients are usually motivated by one of three goals: looking better, feeling better, or performing better—or by some combination of those three. For example, you could tell a ballplayer that if he is less tense, he may be able to throw the ball more easily; you could tell a client struggling with illness that lowering stress can help overall health; and you can tell a client concerned about appearance that people often look more vibrant when they are relaxed and carrying less pain and tension.

Talk to Clients in Words They Understand

In particular, you want to avoid New Age jargon if these words are unfamiliar to your audience. For instance, telling a banker that you want to release the negative vibrations from their third chakra. The same applies to medical terminology. We want to be professional and use the correct terminology, but we also want to avoid sounding so technical that client's haven't a clue what we're talking about. While most clients know what "abs" and "biceps" are, they don't know what the gracilis is or where it's located. We can say, while we're working on an area, "This muscle is your gracilis, and I notice it seems very sore when I touch it. Let me know if I'm working too deeply for your comfort."

Talking with Clients during Sessions

Talking with clients who are on the table takes special sensitivity. During the hands-on work, you want to use a different tone of voice or manner than you would use in normal conversation.

There are a couple of reasons for this extra care. For one, clients on the table are exposed—although protected by draping, they are often naked. Even if they have their clothes on, they are in a passive position. Also, many people have negative judgments about their bodies. Many clients come to you having been told all their lives by their perhaps well-meaning parents, loved ones, and certainly by the culture that they are too fat or too thin, too flabby, too short, too hairy, and so forth. Unless they are unusually self-confident, clients may feel some degree of inadequacy, unhappiness, or even shame about their bodies. You don't want to stand

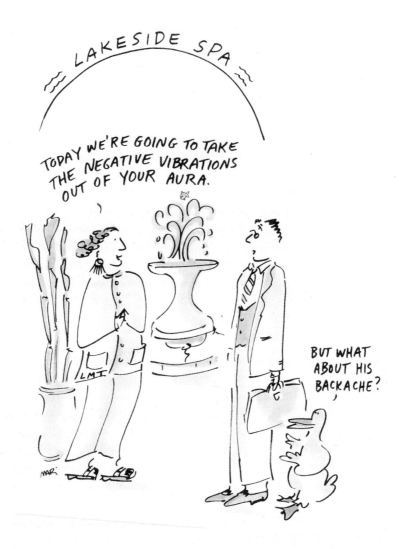

there from the safety of being fully clothed and add to their discouragement with careless words. When clients are on the table, the practitioner's words should be reassuring and positive.

Aside from being sensitive to their vulnerability, you also want to provide a space within which clients can turn off their thinking minds and drop into a state of deep relaxation. In light of those two conditions—wishing to honor clients' vulnerability and allowing a deeply relaxed state—here are some guidelines for talking with clients during the actual session.

Speak As If to a Person Who Is About to Fall Asleep

Use a lighter tone and softer volume than normal conversation. Take care not to say anything that might be upsetting or jarring. Remember that you want to be soothing. If you talk at all, think in terms of using your voice as if it were a third hand.

Keep Your Own Talking to a Minimum

Keep in mind that a yakking practitioner is a major complaint of all clients. A good general policy is to keep your talking to a minimum and keep it focused on the client. (A little chatting can be OK if you sense that the client will think you are rude or cold if you are too silent.) As much as possible, avoid bringing up subjects unrelated to the massage and avoid initiating conversation. Take your cue from the client. Some people, especially those who may be lacking in social interaction because they're retired, widowed, or live alone, *want* to talk. Even so, keep the focus on them. Avoid being too personal about yourself, or asking questions that are too invasive about them. For example, if a client says "I haven't met too many people my age since I moved to town," an appropriate response might be "I noticed on the intake form you live in Wedgewood. They have a really nice senior center there." Asking "Why did you move here, anyway?" is inappropriate.

Don't Ask Questions or Talk in Such a Way That Clients Have to Think to Respond to You

Even though you want to educate your clients, you don't want to engage peoples' brains with long explanations, speeches, or stories. Don't ask them questions that take thought (except very early on in the session before they are deeply relaxed), such as, "How many times have you hurt this foot?" If you need feedback, for instance, to find the right amount of pressure for massage, your goal is still to help them relax as much as possible by keeping questions simple.

You want to limit the amount of time spent in left-brain activity, such as counting or analyzing. Try to ask them questions that involve the right brain, such as questions about feelings or sensations: "How does this feel?" or "How is this pressure?"

Keep Instructions Simple

To avoid getting people to think, you want to keep instructions simple. For example, some people have trouble distinguishing between right and left, and most people, when they are deeply relaxed, have to think to remember which is which. It can be helpful just to tap lightly on the appropriate side and say, "Would you turn over on this side, please? I'll hold the cover while you turn."

Say the Obvious

It's surprising how effective it can be to simply say what seems obvious to you. "You seem to be having a hard time letting go of your right hand. It's been in a fist for much of the session." You don't have to make up fancy explanations or add inter-pretations. Sometimes just bringing a bodily habit or pattern to a client's awareness makes a big difference. It even made a big difference for me, personally, when I was a student and not yet experienced in the ways of massage and didn't yet have much knowledge of anatomy and physiology.

I got my first guitar when I was nine. I used to have chronic neck and shoulder pain, which I jokingly referred to as "guitaritis." When I was in massage school, I was performing in a local venue one night, and the school owner and a bunch of my class-mates came to the show. At the next class, the school owner asked, "Do you have to look at your fingers when you're playing?" When I said no, she said "I don't think you're even aware of it. You are constantly looking to the left (at my fingering hand)." It was really that simple...once she brought it to my attention, every time I played, I started making a conscious effort to stop that habit. It really made a huge difference. Habits become so ingrained that most people are just unaware of them: the woman who always carries her heavy purse on the same shoulder, or her baby on the same hip. Just a gentle reminder to bring it into their consciousness is often all that's needed.

Use Images That Convey the Possibility of Change

You want to let clients know that they can get better, not give the idea they are stuck in an uncomfortable condition. As an example, rather than saying, "This shoulder is like concrete," you can say, "This shoulder joint seems to need more flexibility." Or if an area doesn't have much movement in it, don't say that it looks dead. You can say that it looks "quiet," "asleep," or "as if it wants to move." At the same time, be careful not to promise people you can "fix" whatever is wrong with them.

Find Something Positive to Say About Clients or About How They Are Taking Care of Their Bodies

Compliment your clients for their self-care. They're coming to get a massage or bodywork, aren't they? That's a good start. However, don't comment on how attrac-tive they are. Doing so could sound as if you're sexually interested in them. Speak of "healthy-looking tissue" and legs that "look strong," for example.

Just as your positive words can sink in deeper, so can your negative ones. A friend reports:

➤ *I didn't appreciate when a massage therapist told me, "You have the tightest shoulders I've ever seen." That's a title I didn't want to have.*

Be Creative with Images

Images can help clients stop thinking and let go. Images can touch clients more deeply and stay with the client longer than dry instructions can. For example, you could say, "What if this shoulder were as loose as a rag doll's?" or "Think of your back as a vast Montana sky." Tailor the images to the client's background and interests.

Use Only Gentle Humor

Teasing and sarcasm have a hidden hostility, whereas gentle humor can work well. For instance, to a client with tight shoulders, you could say, "I've been wondering who's been carrying the world around for the rest of us. Looks like it was you."

Of Course, No Flirting

Because of the power difference and the client's vulnerability, any flirting can be intrusive or seen as harassing. No matter what your intention or how innocent a remark or tone of voice may seem, flirting with the client sexualizes the situation and is unethical.

Take Extra Care What You Say When Working Around a Client's Head or Face

When working around a client's head or face, your words can go even more deeply into their unconscious. Because you're so close to clients' ears that it's easy to sound loud and jarring, it's best not to talk at all. If you do speak, use positive words and images. If you say, for instance, "I want to make your neck less tense so you won't have a headache," what may stick in the client's mind is the word "headache." You could say, "It would be great to have more ease here in your neck." Or play with images: "See if you can let your neck be as loose as warm taffy." Keep in mind that work on the face and on the anterior neck may make some people feel claustrophobic, so speak reassuringly.

Be Sympathetic in Your Tone

It's easy for clients to think we're criticizing them. For instance, "You're so tight" can sound like a judgment. We could say instead, "Looks like you've been under some stress," or maybe better, "Have you been under some stress lately?"

Keep the Focus on the Client

When a client says, "My husband makes me mad because he won't wash the dishes," you don't need to add, "Oh, mine, too. Isn't it a drag? The other day, he made me so mad when he...." Clients are paying for your time and attention, not your life story. Sometimes such a remark would be harmless, and sometimes it could be a problem. Suppose your client is an overworked mother who feels that she doesn't get enough personal attention in her life. She may—rightfully—feel intruded on if you take the spotlight away from her.

What could be less relaxing than for someone to command you to "RELAX!"? Instead of doing that, or demanding, "Let this shoulder go," you could say, "I wonder how good it would feel if this shoulder could let go."

Dealing with Common Dilemmas

Certain questions and situations come up over and over in our work. Here are some specific ways to handle them, keeping in mind that our goal is to focus on the client's welfare.

Talkative Clients

If a client is talkative, your main concern is whether the talking is good for the client or not. This is an important point that many massage therapists don't take into account. Clients don't have to be totally quiet in order to receive the most benefit from a massage or bodywork. In fact, some clients unwind by talking, especially during the early parts of a massage.

If you see that talking is making a client more tense or getting in the way of his relaxing, then you need to say something. This is an excellent time to educate and suggest rather than order. Rather than saying, "You'll get more out of your massage if you are quiet," you can say, "Notice what happens to your back (shoulders, neck) as you're talking. It's okay for you to talk, but you may just want to close your eyes and relax if it interferes with receiving the full benefit of the work."

Some clients feel obligated to chat, as if the session were a social interaction. Those clients just need reassurance, "If you really want to talk, that's fine, but this is your hour to relax. You don't need to talk if you'd rather be quiet."

One therapist said "The client was talking so much that it irritated me, so I politely asked her to be quiet." This is a classic case of the therapist making it all about them, instead of all about the client. Practitioners really have no right to ask a client to be quiet unless a client is being abusive or talking loudly enough to disturb other clients. Otherwise, clients should be free to tell you about their grandchildren, recite the Gettysburg address, or talk as much as they want. Your job is to let them know when those activities seem to be getting in the way of *their* relaxation, not yours. Sometimes practitioners are distracted by a client's talking because they feel they must respond, as if it were a normal conversation. Actually, all you need to do is say enough to show that you're listening. "Uh huh... I see." If a client keeps trying to engage you in conversation or if you're newly trained and having a difficult time focusing, then it's okay to say, "It's fine for you to talk, but if I pay too much attention to talking with you, I can't concentrate on doing a good job."

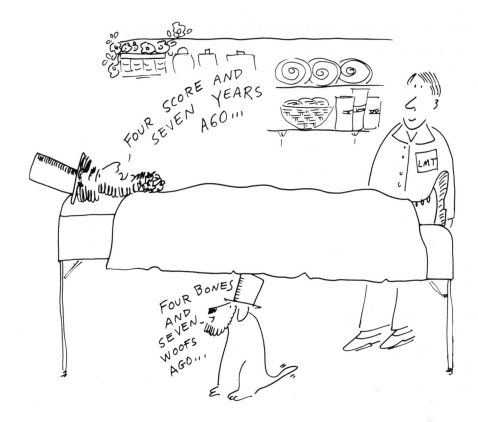

Clients Who Are Emotional or Want Advice

As clients feel comfortable with you, they sometimes talk about their personal lives or ask for advice. Sometimes as they relax, feelings they've held back in their ordinary lives come up, and they may express their anger or sadness. You want to be compassionate with your clients, but sometimes it is difficult to know when you have inappropriately taken on the role of counselor. Let's sort out when you are being true to your role as a manual therapist and when you might be acting too much like a counselor or psychotherapist.

When Clients Want Advice

When a client is in distress, upset, or having trouble, you may feel that you need to do something about it, to fix it. However, your job isn't to fix your clients' personal lives; your job is to create a safe and relaxing atmosphere for them to receive your work.

You can provide a valuable service if you simply listen to your clients. People who are complaining often don't really want advice; they just want to vent. If that helps them to relax, all you have to do is make sympathetic sounds to show that you're listening and being supportive. "Really?" "That's too bad." Any more than that can be overstepping boundaries.

When Clients Are Emotional

Some practitioners are uncomfortable when a client cries; perhaps because they think they must do something about it or stop the client from feeling unhappy. However, bodywork and massage can bring up held-in feelings, and crying can be a helpful release. When clients cry, you don't need to do anything other than perhaps indicate you're aware of their crying: You might want to offer them a tissue or see if they want you to stop working for a minute. There's no need to do anything else; just your presence can be enough of a comfort.

Some practitioners may go too far interpreting the boundaries between psychotherapy and bodywork. They may think that anything outside of massaging muscles isn't their domain, or they become uncomfortable when a client cries or expresses distress about his or her personal life. Here's an example of interpreting our role too narrowly:

➤ *My client had just come back from court, where she had officially ended her 20-year marriage. She was very upset, expressing anger at her ex-husband and also crying. I told her that she might benefit from seeing a counselor and that I wasn't qualified to help her.*

Although there are times when you might need to suggest that a client seek professional counseling, it doesn't take any special training to be a sympathetic ear for clients. If, 6 months after the divorce, this client is still crying and expressing anger at her ex-husband, then you might want to suggest that she seek the services of a counselor. Try to do so in such a way that the client feels supported rather than rejected. "I don't mind your talking about your problems here if it helps you relax, but I wonder if you would also like to see a professional counselor who can support you through this difficult time. I can refer you to someone if you are interested." (Also, consider such a consultation for yourself if you feel overwhelmed when a client cries.)

When Clients May Need Professional Counseling

In general, you might recommend clients seek professional counseling when they seem unable to come out of normal periods of depression or grief by themselves or when they seem overwhelmed by grief or depression—not just feeling sad or unhappy but unable to engage in their lives or work. Also, if clients seem confused

REAL EXPERIENCE

It can be helpful if you personally know a counselor to refer people to, if you've had personal experience with one. It can be disastrous if you give a personal recommendation to a counselor that you don't really know. There is a psychologist in practice very near my office, and I once recommended him to a massage client who had fibromyalgia, and who also had seemed to be in a state of depression lasting for several months. She got an appointment with the counselor, who proceeded to tell her that fibromyalgia does not exist and that it was all in her head. I was mortified, and it was a wake-up call for me not to refer to people I don't actually know. If you do not personally have experience with a counselor, a general recommendation such as "The Pathways Clinic has several counselors on staff," is the best way to go.

—Anonymous, M.T.

about their lives or unable to cope by themselves or if they often ask you for advice, you should recommend that they seek other help. Again, you want to be compassionate and not sound as if you're rejecting them. You might say, "You seem to have a lot of questions about decisions in your life. I can offer you a sympathetic ear, but I don't have the training to help you sort out your marriage (job, relationships). Have you thought about seeing a counselor?"

If you are unsure about how to work with a client because of their emotional needs, consider getting a consultation from a mental health professional as a valuable resource for yourself. Certainly, if clients express feelings of wanting to commit suicide, are engaged in self-destructive behavior, or are being harmed by someone else, you must urge them to seek counseling, and you should immediately get a consultation yourself from a mental health professional to find out the best way to help this client. Depending on the licensing regulations in your state, you may be required to report a client who is in danger of harming himself or herself or someone else.

Clients Asking Personal Questions

Responding appropriately to a client's personal questions about you can be much more complicated than it looks. Although you may respond spontaneously to questions about yourself from friends or acquaintances, knowing how to respond to clients' questions can take more thought. Often, in order to answer a question well, you'll need to understand the reason the client is asking it.

If you answer a personal question without thought, either you could give out more information than the client needs or than you want to reveal or your response could shut out the client in an abrupt way. For instance, a male client asking a female practitioner, "Are you married?" could be asking if she could understand the difficulty he is having with his spouse or could be asking if she is available for a date. If you don't know why a client is asking a question and feel uncomfortable with answering, you might say, "I'm curious why you're asking." To be client centered, you always want to turn the spotlight back on the client—but in a friendly way. You don't want to be abrupt with a client who's just being sociable or trying to connect with you—nor do you want to go into a detailed discussion of your personal life or problems.

If you think the client is looking for support for a difficult marital situation, you could say, "I understand how hard it is to keep clear communication with a partner." If you learn the client is looking for a date, you could simply state your policy that you do not socialize with clients.

Clients may ask personal questions for other reasons also. Some clients feel uncomfortable or impolite if the focus of the session is entirely on them. You can let such clients know that they can relax and concentrate only on the work and on their own concerns. And some clients are merely curious and friendly and have no hidden motive in asking personal questions.

If there is something dramatic or obvious about you that you know clients will ask about—your foot is in a cast, for instance—have your story ready. You don't want to give each client a 15-minute monologue about how your foot got broken. Again, what you want to discern and respond to is why the client is asking the question. A client inquiring about a practitioner's broken foot could be wondering if the wounded practitioner can now more readily identify with their pain, or they may ask, "Even though you are injured, can you still help me today?"

Keeping your privacy and keeping the focus on the client can be difficult for those who live in a small town or are part of a community where people know each other's business. However, if a client brings up something they have learned about you from someone else—"How's your bad back/divorce/leaky roof?"—all you need to do is assure them that all is well, that you are fine and ready to give them your attention and best work.

Clients Asking Questions Outside Your Scope of Practice

When clients ask you a question outside your expertise, it's important to be willing to say, "I don't know." It's a respectable answer. You can say, "Sorry, but I don't have any training in that area, so I don't know how to answer that question." Don't pretend to know or try to bluff your way through answering such a question. Not having to know everything can be freeing for you, and your clients will appreciate the honesty of an "I don't know." It educates them about what you do know and what your areas of expertise are. Showing your clients that you honor your limits helps them trust you. Clients won't usually be dismayed or shocked that you don't know everything; they just move on to their next concern.

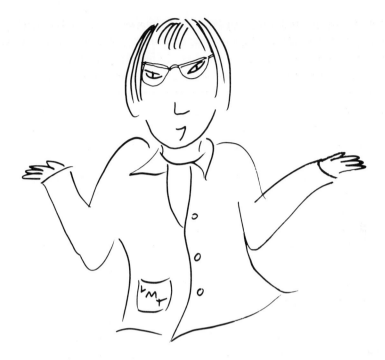

Feeling that you have to know the answer to every question either directly or remotely related to the body can make your work stressful and stifle your curiosity. You could find yourself falling back on rote answers. "The way to work with this kind of knee is to do X." Having to know can make you miss out on what's going on right here, right now, in front of you with this client.

Clients Who Are Demanding

Clients who seem critical, demanding, or controlling can be a challenge; you don't want to take their behavior personally. Avoid getting into negative countertransference. Keep in mind that clients may be acting out of fear that stems from past trauma. Although you may never know what clients' histories are, demanding or critical clients are often communicating that it is hard for them to feel safe. Their message may be that they are not sure you are going to pay enough attention to their care. If you respond to their demands with impatience or irritation, you could be proving their assumptions true.

It is better to try to let them know you're doing your best. "Is there anything I can do to make you feel more at ease?" If a client persists in being demanding, you can say gently, "I feel like you're not comfortable, and I want this to be a good experience for you. I hope you will let me know what else I can do." Your honesty and openness may help the client trust that your intentions are good.

It's rare for clients to express directly that they were unsatisfied with your work and that they don't want to work with you again. However, if that happens, it's best to end the relationship in a way that doesn't blame either of you. You could say, "I'm sorry that you're not happy with the massage (or bodywork session). For some reason, we just don't work well together." Or "Perhaps my style of working isn't what you're looking for. I can give you the names of some other therapists in the area."

Setting Limits

The ability to set limits gracefully and effectively is vital to our professional lives, especially for those in private practice.

If clients don't know what the boundaries are, it's difficult for them to feel safe with you. Although we may not think of setting limits as a skill that we need to learn, the reality is that our limit-setting skills need to be practiced and polished as much as our hands-on skills.

If clients don't know what the boundaries are, it's difficult for them to feel safe with you.

If you have an employer, usually they are the ones who handle such things as setting and collecting fees (and tips), punctuality, and sexual inappropriateness (although this is not always the case). You may not have many opportunities to set limits yourself, but you can learn by observing what works and what doesn't in how your employer sets limits both with you and with clients.

Here's an example about how being unclear about expectations can cause problems for both you and your client. A colleague reports:

➤ *I had a client who raved about my work and said he was going to tell all his friends about my "miracle work." Well, that kind of praise went to my head, and I let it interfere with my judgment. When he started coming late and missing appointments without calling, I didn't say anything to him or charge him for the missed time. In fact, I even altered personal plans to create a time slot for him—and he didn't show for the appointment!*

➤ *I know that I would have set limits sooner with another client, but I was caught up in being "the miracle worker," and that wasn't good for either of us. Every time I didn't set good boundaries, he pushed another limit. I wish I could say that I started setting limits, but the truth is that he just stopped making appointments. I did him a disservice by not being clear about boundaries and expectations.*

Setting Limits Gracefully

The most awkward and pesky dilemmas, particularly for those who are self-employed, are how to deal with clients who sexualize the situation and how to maintain boundaries around time and fees. Knowing what to do with clients who make passes or who act sexually inappropriate is discussed in Chapter 8. The following sections discuss some ways to make setting limits about time and money easier for you. Of course, you may want to rephrase these responses in words that feel natural to you.

Be Clear About Expectations in Advance

This point can't be stressed enough. It's much easier and less awkward to set limits when you know you've been clear with the client about your policies from the beginning. It's a good idea to get in the habit of starting to educate clients during the first phone call about your fee policies, time policies, and, if necessary, the nonsexual nature of your work. For instance, assuming this is your policy, make sure you always say, "If you need to cancel, please let me know at least 24 hours ahead of time so I have time to schedule someone else; otherwise, I'll have to charge you for the session." If you make it a habit, then you don't have to wonder later on whether you've told a client about the policy. About time policies, you can say, "Your appointment will start at 4 p.m.; please be on time so that we can have a full hour to work together."

First sessions need to include time not only for gathering information from the client but also for educating the client about your professional standards—in written form and verbal form. That can include policies about late arrival, notice to cancel, payment options (such as whether you take credit cards or checks), confidentiality, and your right to refuse to work with a client who acts inappropriately. Find policies that you're comfortable with, be clear about them with your clients from the beginning, and then follow through as necessary. Having your policies in writing and asking clients to sign or initial forms is a good idea. Since the form they sign will be remaining in your office, it's a good idea to have a copy you can give to clients. That way, you can avoid the situation of clients saying "I wasn't informed I'd be charged for a missed appointment!"

Be Careful About Your Tone

When you have to set a limit, be matter of fact and even sympathetic but not apologetic. "I understand that you couldn't make your appointment last week because you decided to go out of town. Unfortunately, since you didn't let me know you weren't coming in, I have to follow my policy and charge you for that session." Avoid taking a parental or judgmental tone with a client. ("You need to be more considerate of my time.")

The first year that I was in business for myself, I had one other therapist working in the office. I hate to say it, but I did not have an official cancellation policy. Whenever anyone cancelled at the last minute, or just failed to show up, we drew a line through the appointment and used "LMC (last minute cancellation)" or "NSNC (no show no call)" abbreviations to indicate the situation. At the end of the first year, I counted the income we had lost due to these incidents, and it amounted to over $8,000! I was shocked. The first thought that popped into my head was "that's a month in Europe!" I ended up handling this situation by taking several actions. I added an official cancellation policy to our intake forms, put a sign on the front desk, put it on our website, and sent out an announcement in our monthly newsletter. After that rude awakening, I immediately put a place for clients to sign on the intake form acknowledging that they have been informed of our cancellation policy and agree to abide by it.

Speak in Terms of Your General Policy Rather Than Personalizing the Limit

You can depersonalize what you say by referring to your general rules: "It's my policy to charge when a session is cancelled within 24 hours unless the client had an emergency."

Practice What You Would Say in Various Situations

Some practitioners have a difficult time setting limits. Remember that setting limits is a skill just like learning massage strokes; it takes practice to become a pro. To become more comfortable and more effective with limit setting, it's a good idea to practice with nonclient friends and relatives; try out what you would say in various situations.

It may sound silly, like play-acting, but **role-playing** is a great way to hone your skills. Even though you may feel mentally prepared to deal with a situation, it helps to say the words out loud. Usually, the same feelings that you would have in the actual situation—awkwardness, fear, and so forth—will arise, even though it's not a real-life situation. Also, your colleague can give you useful feedback about the effectiveness of your tone, words, and demeanor.

Role-playing:
Usually, a structured exercise in which students or colleagues take a role—for instance, as client or practitioner—and act out a specific situation as a way of becoming more comfortable with handling the situation in real life.

Here's a success story from Brian Thayer, LMT, a massage therapist, who at the time was a recent graduate of a massage therapy school that uses role-playing. (If you're out of school or your school doesn't offer role-playing, you can set up your own role-playing with willing friends or colleagues.)

➤ *My first paying client turned out to be a great learning experience. I was really nervous beforehand. After the intake process, I left the room to give him privacy, saying, "Please feel free to get undressed to a level that you are comfortable with and get on the table under this sheet face up." When I said "under this sheet," I put my hand under the top sheet and turned it over slightly.*

When I returned, I knocked on the door, opened it, and found my client lying face down, completely nude on top of the sheet. As if I wasn't nervous enough!

I took a deep breath and said, "Oops, let me step out of the room while you get under the top sheet and turn face up, please." As I stepped out of the room and closed the door, my calm, centered state escaped me. Taking a deep breath, I knocked on the door again and entered. This time he was under the sheet lying face up, but asked, grabbing the sheet, "Is this really necessary?" My reply was, "Actually, I use proper draping for all my sessions. It is the law that clients must be draped."

I was so pleased that the right words came out of my mouth without a second thought! What made the difference was that I had role-played that very situation with a fellow student, saying what I would say when or if a situation like that came up. They say practice makes perfect: for me, practice made permanent.

Most of us come into this work because we want to help people; an important part of how we help is by setting clear boundaries. Clients feel safer and practitioners are more at ease when we all know what to expect and where the limits are.

The Right Words

Although our work is centered on nonverbal communication, our words make a difference. We want them to enhance our hands-on work and make our jobs easier. Because each client and each situation is unique, there will always be challenges. No matter how long we are in practice, there will always be times when we find ourselves searching for the right words and occasionally stumbling. Our goal is to know that what we say makes a difference and to keep looking for words that connect with our clients.

Questions for Reflection

1. You have had two previous sessions with a client. On the day of his third appointment, he or she didn't show up. Practicing with a colleague or friend, put into your own words what you would say or ask when you call this client.

2. Have you ever been a client, trying to settle in and relax on the table with a massage therapist or bodyworker who talked in such a way that it was hard for you to stay relaxed? What could that practitioner have done differently to enhance your relaxation?

3. A client calls at the last minute to cancel an appointment because he or she "just can't get away from work right now." This client canceled at the last minute once before. At that time, even though you had explained your

policy of needing 24 hours' notice, you didn't charge him for the missed session. What would you say to him or her now?

4. Is there a situation involving limit setting that you dread dealing with? How can you make the situation easier for yourself?

5. Imagine you, the practitioner, are a pregnant woman, just starting to show. (You don't have to be pregnant or even a woman to imagine this.) Your client begins to ask you questions about your due date, marital status, and how you feel. How do you keep the conversation client centered—how do you steer it back to the client? What underlying concerns might the client have about how your pregnancy would affect your professional work and relationship with him or her? How would you find out what those concerns might be, and how would you address them?

---

thePoint To learn more about the concepts discussed in this chapter, visit http://thePoint .lww.com/Allen-McIntosh4e

CHAPTER 7

Sexual Boundaries: Protecting Our Clients

Many of us are led to this work for high-minded reasons. For many, there's a wish to bring greater ease into the lives of others. Some even see this work as a sacred calling, a way to heal the soul and enliven the spirit. But despite the good intentions we bring to our sessions, because we're working closely with the physical body, we can't avoid the murkiness and confusion of sexual issues.

Sometimes clients are sexually attracted to their practitioners. Sometimes practitioners, like any other professional, are attracted to their clients. The intimacy of our work can be confusing to both client and practitioner. We are touching people, often with a tenderness and gentle attentiveness that is almost like a lover's. When the professional boundaries are clear, it can be wonderfully healing for the client. When they aren't, it can be harmful or even disastrous.

The honest pleasure of sensuality is part of the profession, but the dark possibilities of seduction and exploitation are lurking in the background. Whether we are in private practice or work for someone else, how do we keep our sessions safe for our clients and avoid even subtle boundary violations and misunderstandings about sexual boundaries?

To begin with, we need to be able to talk honestly with others about these issues. When there isn't enough dialogue, we don't learn from one another. During the time I spent on our state board, participating in disciplinary hearings of therapists who had been accused of wrong-doing, and during the time I spent doing research for this book, I realized how complex and painful the stories were from both clients and practitioners. I heard of well-meaning and presumably well-trained practitioners who had stumbled into tangled, destructive situations that might have been avoided had they known the warning signs and acted on them.

> *The honest pleasure of sensuality is part of the profession, but the dark possibilities of seduction and exploitation are lurking in the background. How do we keep our sessions safe for our clients and avoid even subtle boundary violations and misunderstandings about sexual boundaries?*

- A male massage therapist ends sessions by kissing female clients on the forehead, a seemingly small gesture that could nevertheless be seen as offensive and invasive (and did in fact end with a complaint and disciplinary hearing resulting in sanctions).
- A female practitioner works close to a client's genitals and is accused of sexual harassment.
- A bodyworker who became sexually involved with a client only later sees how harmful the relationship was to the client (and to her, ultimately).

The emotions in these situations run deep for both client and practitioner. Even if falsely accused of violating a client, a practitioner's distress can be long lasting. And because of the power difference between client and practitioner, the effect on the client when sexual boundaries are crossed, whether intentional or not, can be deeply damaging.

Transference, Countertransference, and Sexual Boundaries

It is in the arena of sexual violations, the most potentially destructive of violations, that we see the powerful protection that professional boundaries can provide. Here's where being sensitive to boundaries and to the effects of transference and countertransference really pays off, steering us clear of harmful mistakes.

The situations described in this chapter present examples of how transference and countertransference can cloud our own judgment and that of our clients.

Positive Transference: Crushes

Sometimes a practitioner is bewildered or even put off when a client develops a strong crush on him or her. In Chapter 4, practitioners are warned not to take crushes personally, not to assume that a crush means that the client wants to have a romantic relationship. It's so common for a client to have a crush, and so easily misinterpreted, that it's worthwhile to explore crushes further: how do they happen and how should we handle them?

It's not unusual for people to develop crushes on any professional who works closely with them, especially when the practitioner is kind to them when they feel vulnerable. For example, clients often become attached to their divorce lawyers, and patients often idolize compassionate physicians.

We have to keep in mind the special intimacy of a bodywork session. Clients bring all kinds of tender longings, old hurts, and broken hearts to their sessions. And there we are—the picture of kindliness, warmth, and selfless giving. We can seem to be the perfect parent, friend, or confidante they have always wanted. It's easy for clients to "fall in love" with us.

Even though there may be a hint of sexual interest, crushes are usually not the same as grown-up feelings of sexual attraction. These crushes are more similar to the kinds of feelings a third grader has for her favorite teacher or the adoration a young boy might have for the star high-school athlete.

Here are some suggestions for dealing with crushes so that both client and practitioner are protected.

Don't Take It Personally

There's no need to be either dismayed or flattered when a client has an innocent crush on you. You don't want to let your awareness of a client's feelings diminish your warmth and friendliness.

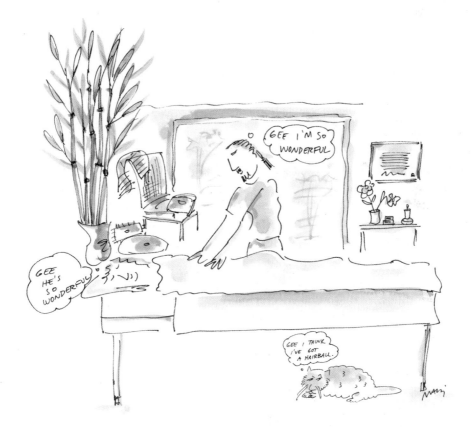

Innocent crushes need to be treated as a sign of the client's trust. The client has judged you to be safe, and you shouldn't make any more of it than that. It can be flattering to have someone wide-eyed over you, hanging on your every word and laughing at your jokes. But you can't let it go to your head. You have to remember that clients have special feelings about you because of the role that you take on, not because of who you are in everyday life. Do your best to remain centered and respectful with clients who have crushes on you.

If a client's attachment to you is upsetting to you, recognize that the problem lies with your discomfort, not the client's feelings (assuming that the client isn't overstepping boundaries). Talk with a trusted teacher or even a mental health counselor to help turn the experience into a healthy learning, one for both you and your client.

Don't Embarrass the Client

A colleague reports:

> ➤ *When I had just graduated from massage therapy school, I was concerned when one of my clients seemed to have a crush on me. I could tell she just adored me. It was kind of flattering, but even though she didn't make any suggestions and I knew that she was happily married, it made me uncomfortable. I wasn't sure whether I should talk to her about it or not, so I talked to my consultant who helps me with problems related to client dynamics. He said not to say anything to her and just to keep focusing on giving her a good massage. That was good advice. Gradually, the crush seemed to dissipate, and we had a solid and warm professional relationship. She was a client for many years.*

As you can see, there was no need for the practitioner to talk with the client about her crush. If he'd mentioned it, she might have felt embarrassed or patronized, which wouldn't have been helpful in resolving her feelings for the practitioner.

Protect Yourself from Inappropriate Clients

There are times when you do need to protect yourself. Don't assume a crush is innocent if a client touches you inappropriately, makes a pass at you, or asks you for a date. You need to set firm limits with such clients. First, make it clear that such behavior isn't appropriate and that you don't date clients. Then, if you feel comfortable continuing the session or continuing to work with this client, you may do so. However, if the client seems disrespectful, you just don't trust them, or you feel uneasy, you can tell them the session is over and that they're not welcome as a client again, and then immediately leave the treatment room.

Take Care with Boundaries

Clients who have crushes sometimes invite their practitioners to socialize with them. What they often want is not the usual give-and-take of a social relationship but a continuation of the therapeutic relationship in which the focus is on them.

Boundary Lessons

When I was attending massage school years ago, there was no dress code at our school and everybody seemed to be pretty casual. One day I traded massage with a male student I had not worked with before. He was face up on the table, and as I was working on his leg at the side of the table, bending forward, and he said "Nice boobs." I took my hands off him and said "That is totally inappropriate!" He said "I know it is, and I didn't mean anything by it. The fact is, when you're bent over me, I'm getting a clear view. I just wanted to point that out, because you need to be careful when you're working on clients." I took a look at what I was wearing and realized he was right, even though I had not been attempting to dress "sexy." I started paying closer attention to myself in the mirror every morning, bending forward, making sure I wasn't exposing cleavage. It was a good lesson and I'm grateful it was a fellow student that pointed it out before I got into professional practice.

—A.O., LMT

It's not a good idea to see any clients outside the office setting—this is particularly true of clients with crushes. If you're tempted to do so, be honest with yourself. Are you enjoying the crush? Are you hoping to flirt or take it further? If a client with a crush on you asked you to a party and you showed up, couldn't that give the message that you're interested in the client? You have to respect the vulnerability of your clients by keeping the relationship within professional boundaries.

Positive Countertransference: "Special" Clients

Feeling that one client is exceptional and different from your other clients, finding yourself really looking forward to their appointments, wanting to rush into dating that client, and thinking that others wouldn't understand the "special" feelings the two of you have—all these are warning signs. Intense feelings about clients are generally indications of countertransference. When there is that adolescent sense that the intensity of the attraction or the specialness of the relationship between the two of you justifies breaking the rules, it is a red flag.

Of course, all your clients are special and need to be appreciated for their uniqueness. But being overwhelmed with attraction to a client or intensely identifying with a client is different from having compassion for or even loving your clients. A sense of specialness about a client is a problem when it leads you to treat that client differently from others, when you feel that the client is so special that you don't have to adhere to the usual boundaries when working with him or her. In the therapeutic relationship, this can be traumatizing for both parties, as in the following story told by a colleague:

➤ *A woman related that during the course of seeing a bodyworker for many months, she developed an intense transference—she was deeply infatuated with her practitioner. She also felt that the practitioner was very drawn to her and that the practitioner had lost objectivity. The relationship developed into an inappropriate situation in which, under the guise of therapy, the therapist had touched the client's breasts and genitals during several sessions. The client ended up feeling emotionally and physically seduced and damaged. Her confused feelings of shame and guilt were so powerful that she didn't discuss this relationship with anyone, until several years later, when she was able to talk with a counselor about it.*

No matter how seductive the client or how equal you feel the relationship is, practitioners are responsible for keeping good professional boundaries. It's important to remember that your relationships with clients are never equal and that you can damage your clients if you act on inappropriate feelings. When clients have crushes on you, those feelings can be part of a positive therapeutic experience if boundaries are kept. If you are tempted to take the relationship further, get a consultation from a mental health professional to help you sort out your feelings. If you are at risk of violating boundaries, you need to dismiss the client—*before* you do something wrong.

Dating an Ex-Client

Given the dynamics of transference and countertransference, you can see the problems with dating an ex-client. Is it ever ethical or safe for the client? The answer is, it depends. It depends on the professional relationship, the intensity of the transference, how emotionally stable the client is, how emotionally stable the practitioner is, how long the therapeutic relationship lasted (was it one or two massages or a long-term relationship), and how much time has elapsed since the therapeutic work. The most important questions are whether the transference and countertransference issues are resolved, and that's a complex issue to gauge, and whether the therapist is remaining in compliance with the law.

Remember, our clients are not obligated to adhere to the code of ethics and standards of practice as put forth by the massage board—we are the one who are obligated to adhere to them. The responsibility is on us.

The rules of many state boards have requirements about dating clients after ending the professional relationship, usually 6 months to 1 year. Practitioners need to check with the licensing laws in their states and the ethical guidelines of their professional organizations. Of course, if you work for someone else, you need to know your employer's rules about dating ex-clients.

The reason for delaying social interaction after concluding the professional relationship is to make sure that neither the client nor the practitioner is still caught up in the rosy glow of transference and countertrans-ference. There needs to be time for reality to set in.

Regardless of what the board rules allow, however, there may be clients that you could never ethically date. There are some circumstances that would make the transference so strong that a sexual relationship would never be appropriate with the client. For instance, if a client has been helped out of great physical or emotional pain by a practitioner, he or she might always see that practitioner as a larger-than-life hero. A practitioner who is able to provide relief from pain when all other methods have failed may always seem like a savior to that client. Also, any circumstances that would make a client look up to a practitioner may help create a relationship in which there can never be equal power—for instance, if a bodyworker is a teacher or is well-known in the community.

However, in some circumstances, dating an ex-client might not bring problems. For example, if a bodyworker is in a health spa and only saw a client once, it is more likely that a strong transference did not develop. Even then, the bodyworker would have to consider how dating an ex-client would affect their reputation and the rep-utation of the profession.

> ➤ *A former client with a crush on his bodyworker asked her for a date. Because she was able to honestly say that she never dates ex-clients, he was able to save face and continue feeling positive about their work together. Suppose the bodyworker had refused him and he knew of other ex-clients she had dated? Suppose she had accepted and had developed a relationship with him, and it had ended in quarrels? Aside from the personal pain on both sides, unhappy ex-clients are not good for public relations, and that's magnified in a small town or rural area.*

You also have to consider that if present clients heard that you were dating an ex-client, it might interfere with their therapeutic relationship with you.

Practitioners of **emotionally-oriented body-work** that often evokes deep transference should give serious consideration before beginning to date an ex-client. The possibility for taking ad-vantage of a former client's transference is strong. Practitioners of such work are often walking a dan-gerously thin line between manual therapy and psychotherapy—something that is *not* within our scope of practice. Taking continuing education in such work may be valuable for having more insight into the psychological dynamics of the therapeu-tic relationship, but it does not mean you have a license to practice counseling or psychology.

Emotionally-oriented bodywork: It is also called psychologically oriented bodywork: Manual therapy that is based on the idea that physical tension and restriction are related to unconscious patterns of holding that the client has adopted, often early in life, to cope with his or her emotional environment. The practitioner facilitates the client in releasing these holdings for the greater emotional and physical well-being of the client.

In any circumstances, you must take into account the emotional stability of the client. For instance, does the client have solid self-esteem, or are they prone to depression, easily influenced, in crisis, or facing any other situation that would make them emotionally fragile? Some clients may not be able to see themselves as equals with their practitioner.

Whether to date an ex-client isn't a decision to make lightly. Even if you are certain that you're not taking advantage of a client, just by dating an ex-client, you're opening yourself to scrutiny by your colleagues and clients and possibly risking damage to your reputation and that of the profession.

Dual Relationships

You would think that the more someone knows you, the less likely it is that they would misread your intentions. However, the opposite is often true.

Dual relationships can cause problems with sexual boundaries; in such relationships, the boundaries are already blurred. Working with people you know in some other way, doing trades, or working with people who share a community with you may sometimes lead to confusion about sexual boundaries. You would think that the more someone knows you, the less likely it is that they would misread your intentions. However, the opposite is often true.

Here's how the dynamic of transference affected a trade between two colleagues:

➤ *Sally, a massage therapist who had been sexually abused by her father, agreed to do a trade with Jim for sessions in his form of emotionally-oriented bodywork. As the trade went on, transference factors caused her to unconsciously see Jim as a father figure. At the same time, the bodywork was bringing up memories and feelings about her abuse. To fulfill her side of the trade, she gave Jim a massage every other week. On a deep level, it was confusing to Sally. It was too hard to relate to Jim as both her therapist and a client whose naked body she was touching. For instance, she began to wonder if Jim was sexually interested in her, even though he seemed happily married. Although she discussed her concerns with Jim and believed him when he said he wasn't attracted to her, she realized she was too uncomfortable with the trade and ended it.*

Trades can make it difficult to maintain clear and clean boundaries. Although they can work out well, it usually takes extra effort to make sure they do. Practitioners doing emotionally-oriented work or deep structural work should probably avoid trades for bodywork, especially those that are ongoing. The confusion brought about by transference and countertransference makes such trades potentially problematic.

The same confusion can occur if you are working with someone who is part of a "family" group that you're in—for instance, you're both serious students of the same yoga teacher, you're in the same Buddhist community, or you're members of the same church. When you're working with such a person, you need to be alert to the negative transference about "family" that can get projected onto you because of your mutual association with that group; not everyone has good memories of family. Even though whatever group you both belong to may be spiritual and well-intentioned, your client may have buried in their unconscious the idea that "family" means abuse and may associate you with that negative picture.

Secrets

You are headed for trouble any time you are doing something with a client or even having a feeling about a client that you want to keep secret (we are not talking about the client's confidentiality here) or that you would not share with your colleagues. When you feel that desire for secrecy, the best thing to do is get it out in the open (without violating the client's confidentiality, of course). As hard as it may seem, share your secret with a teacher or consultant. It could be that there is no reason for you to feel uncomfortable. Or it could be that you need help with the client before the situation turns into an even more difficult problem.

Clients Who Have Been Sexually Abused

As we have seen, transference can lead clients to unconsciously associate us with past authority figures. This transference can be especially charged if a client was sexually abused as a child.

When children are sexually abused, the abuser is often a member of the family—perhaps a father, a mother, or an older relative, or an authority figure they trusted, such as a teacher or priest. Abused children can rightfully feel betrayed: someone who was supposed to be protecting them and taking care of them has taken advantage of them. Sometimes those feelings of betrayal and mistrust linger, usually on an unconscious level, even after the individual becomes an adult. Although it is not true of every individual who was sexually abused, some clients who were abused as children will transfer those feelings of mistrust onto anyone who is a caregiver or an authority figure, which can include massage and bodywork practitioners.

Because of these associations, some clients come to sessions with an underlying (and usually unconscious) distrust of the practitioner and perhaps with the expectation that the practitioner will, at the least, not take good care of them and, at the most, exploit them.

Other kinds of behavior may be seen in clients who have been sexually abused. They may be hyper-alert to signs of danger or seduction and, therefore, more likely to misread a careless word or gesture. They may have a distorted sense of what appropriate boundaries are: they may be blind to a truly dangerous situation when a therapist is being inappropriate or may even test the practitioner by being seductive themselves.

Interactions with sexually-abused clients can be complicated if the practitioner has also experienced such abuse. Practitioners who have a history of being abused can have the same kinds of distorted perceptions that clients do. They can assume that a client has sexual intentions when he does not, or they can fail to respond adequately when a client actually is being offensive. Practitioners who have been sexually abused may also be unable to see their own seductiveness or inappropriateness with a client. Crossing boundaries may unconsciously feel comfortable and familiar to them.

Here are a couple of examples of what can happen:

➤ *Before the session begins, a female massage therapist announces to a new male client who has not shown any signs of acting inappropriately that she has pepper spray that she will use if he gets out of line.*

➤ *A male bodyworker flirts with all his female clients and often accepts social invitations from them. He doesn't initiate the invitations, but justifies it in his own mind with "they asked, so why not?"*

In the first example, the practitioner is being overly self-protective; in the second, the practitioner cannot see the violations he is committing. (Of course, practitioners can overreact or commit violations without having a history of being abused.)

Because of the potential for confusion and missteps, the safest way to avoid making serious errors with clients is to stick to accepted boundaries and provide a stable framework. We may never know what history a client brings to the table, and it is not our place to ask clients whether they have been sexually abused. However, we are safer if we treat *all* clients with the care that we would use if we knew that they were in need of special sensitivity.

Working with Clients Who Have Been Sexually Abused

Statistics on sexual abuse vary. Some say that at least one in three women and one in twelve men have been sexually abused. Because so many people have experienced sexual abuse that you probably cannot avoid working with someone who has, it is a good idea to be educated about how to work with such clients. Also, if you are in private practice and you have a client who is actively dealing with issues of sexual abuse in psychotherapy, you need to contact the client's psychotherapist (with the client's written permission) to make sure that the work you are doing is beneficial to the client. Consulting with that psychotherapist or another mental health professional also is very helpful.

REAL EXPERIENCE

When I was in massage school, I was working in the student clinic with a female client. It had been impressed on the class that male therapists needed to exercise extra diligence when working with female clients, and that some females would not be comfortable having a male therapist. The client was face up on the table, and I asked her if she would like to have her abdominals massaged; I never did that (and still don't, 15 years later) without asking permission. She said yes, so I put a towel drape over her breasts, and started pulling the sheet down from under the towel to expose her abdominal area. I had not even gotten as far as her navel when she loudly screamed "That's far enough!" She yelled so loudly that the clinic supervisor came to the door to see if there was a problem. It almost made me afraid to ask any other clients about abdominal work. I've never had another experience like that—thankfully—but it scared the daylights out of me. We never know what's going on inside someone's head or what will set them off.

—C.A., LMBT

Not every client who has been sexually abused is in need of counseling. However, if you have reason to believe that a client needs to see a psychotherapist—for instance, a regular client seems depressed or self-destructive—you can suggest counseling. While you may provide your regular massage therapy services to such a client, never attempt to delve into a client's sexual abuse issues on your own. Such work takes experience and training. For your own safety—for instance, to avoid being falsely accused of sexual harassment by an overly vigilant client—it's a good idea to seek outside help with the psychological dynamics of the relationship.

All manual therapists need to educate themselves by reading relevant literature and attending workshops on working with clients who have been sexually abused. On rare occasions, such clients have flashbacks during the session: they experience the memory of the abuse as if it is happening in the moment. Education can prepare you to deal with such situations and can help you feel more confident with other signs of sexual abuse.

Most of the effects of sexual abuse that you will encounter are not dramatic. The signs of abuse that you will see most often are usually less obvious. As noted previously, such clients may be more wary and slow to trust. They may seem controlling or demanding. They may have a more difficult time letting go and relaxing. Or they may be seductive. (Of course, not every client who is wary, controlling, tense, or seductive has been abused.)

There are simple ways that you can help sensitive clients feel safer. Of course, these precautions are valuable in working with any client.

Don't Push Clients

If clients seem numb in a particular area, don't push them to feel it. Work somewhere else. If a client shares a memory of abuse but doesn't have a complete picture, don't push him or her to remember it. Remembering an incident of abuse isn't necessary to healing, and it can often be retraumatizing for the client. Leave the treatment of sexual abuse issues to those who have extensive training and experience.

Stay Sympathetic but Objective

If a client tells you about an experience of being sexually abused, be a sympathetic listener but be careful about sharing your opinion or experience. For instance, talking about what a bad person the perpetrator was is not a good idea. If the perpetrator was also someone the client felt close to, he or she may have mixed and confusing feelings about the person, including loyalty or affection.

Make Sure Clients Have a Voice

Because of transference and feelings of dependency, clients often don't speak up when you're making them uncomfortable. This is especially true when the discomfort is around a sexual issue. Even if the client is an acquaintance or a colleague and even if the person is usually assertive in the outside world, once in the role of client, she or he can have a hard time saying no.

> ➤ *A successful businesswoman receiving a massage in a spa thought that the practitioner was working too close to her genitals. She didn't think the massage therapist, an older woman, was making sexual advances, but she was still uncomfortable. In the business world, the businesswoman had a diplomatic but straightforward style of dealing with people and gave critical feedback easily. In the role of client, however, she said nothing but never went back to that therapist.*

It can help clients voice their feelings if you demonstrate in many ways your interest in hearing how they feel and what they have to say. Be sure to ask clients to let you know if anything you do makes them uncomfortable. Let clients know that they can always ask you to stop, even if they do not have a reason that seems rational (to you) and even if they feel that they are being rude by doing so. Avoid the appearance of dominating a client.

Other Cautions and Red Flags

There are a number of other areas where it makes sense to be cautious and to think of the potential for misinterpretation by a vulnerable client.

Professional Appearance

Short shorts, tank tops, and cleavage are for off-hours. Don't dress as if you're going out on a date to the club or to the beach. You can be comfortable and still look like a reliable professional. Basically, you want to wear clean, neat, loose clothes that don't draw attention to your body.

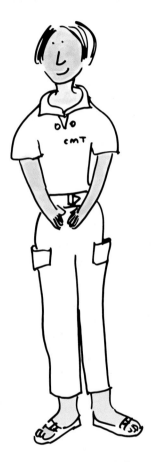

In some parts of the country, especially small towns and rural areas, a purple Mohawk, visible tattoos and unusual facial rings, such as nose or eyebrow rings, raise other people's eyebrows and make you work harder to convince them that you are safe and professional. Let your work show people how special you are—not your jewelry or body art.

Language

You need to be careful that your language isn't even remotely suggestive or flirta-tious. For instance, it's best not to tell clients, "Take off your clothes." That sounds

Many massage therapists work barefooted. In fact, Ashiatsu practitioners perform massage with their bare feet. The client usually (but not always) knows when they request an Ashiatsu session what it is going to be. However, for those who aren't practicing that, consider how that appears to the client. If you walked into the doctor's office and the physician and nursing staff were in their bare feet, would you have confidence in them, or would you think they were flaky and unprofessional? If you made an appointment with a licensed professional, such as an attorney or accountant, would you have confidence in them if you arrived to find them dressed in short shorts, a tank top, and in their bare feet? One therapist stated in an online forum that she stopped working in her bare feet when she got a client who had a foot fetish. You may not think that people are going to be sexually excited by your feet, but it happens.

like an order, and it is too close to words that would be used in a sexual encounter. Instead, say something such as, "I'll leave the room for a few minutes so that you can get ready for the session. Please undress to your level of comfort and get under the covers face up."

We should keep in mind that people who have never had a massage—and some who have—may not know what clothing to remove, or that they don't have to remove something they feel uncomfortable removing. It is up to us to educate them, and to bear with whatever the client feels comfortable with. I personally had a rodeo cowboy as a client for several years. He wanted his back massaged, and that was it. Even though I discussed with him that his glutes were involved in his back pain, and that the whole body was connected, he was not comfortable with that. He got his massage wearing his Levi's, his cowboy boots, and a huge silver belt buckle. That was what he wanted, so I just worked with it the best I could.

Some women don't want to remove their bra. You should ask if you may unsnap it to work on their back, or pull the straps down to work on their shoulders, and tell them that it's their choice. We should never assume that it's okay and just do it without asking. If a client has left their underwear on, for example, you may say "Is it okay if I tuck the sheet into your underwear and move it down a little so I may work on your lower back?" Most people will be fine with that. If someone is not, don't make them feel uncomfortable about it and just work through their clothing.

Choose your words carefully when you say anything about a client's body. Even saying, "Why do you criticize your body? You look great!" can sound overly personal or suggestive. You might sometimes want to compliment a client who seems to have a negative body image. When clients make unflattering comments about their bodies, you can say something general such as, "Gosh, women (or just people) are so hard on themselves about how they look." To be sure you avoid being heard as expressing sexual attraction, however, you're better off avoiding all comments about how you think the client's body looks aesthetically. Besides having the potential to be seen as a come-on, making such a remark puts you in the position of being an expert on how bodies should look, which, of course, you're not. Avoid sounding critical or judgmental, as well. Don't make comments like "Don't you regret getting that tattoo?" or "I could never get a hole in my ear like that."

Draping

Draping is always a good idea. In most regulated states, it is also the law. When in doubt, go for more cover rather than for less. It's respectful to the client's privacy and a way to protect yourself from misunderstandings.

You will sometimes get clients who don't want to be draped. Even if it is not required by law, it can be one of your personal boundaries. You can say "It's my policy to drape all clients. I'm not comfortable working on undraped people." Draping is for us, as much as the client. What if you had a client on the table who had the largest breasts you've ever seen, or a penis that reaches down to their midthigh? Are you really going to be able to avoid staring at that? Draping is for the modesty, comfort, and safety of the client—*and for ours*.

REAL EXPERIENCE

I was in a student massage clinic that was being conducted in a big, open classroom many years ago. There were no privacy curtains; the people receiving massage would go into the bathroom, disrobe and wrap in the top sheet, and then come out and get on the table. There were about 25 tables set up with a student and a client at each one. A male student was giving me a massage. I was face up on the table, very relaxed with my eyes closed, when I suddenly felt the sheet sliding off my body, totally exposing me. The student quickly grabbed it and covered me, but he was so mortified, I thought he was going to have a heart attack on the spot. He was wearing a lotion holster, and when he bent over me, it snagged the sheet and pulled it off me. Most of the people in the room were focused on their own massage, and I don't think many people saw it happen. He later told me that he felt like he was taking a driver's test and passed a stopped school bus! He had no intent to expose me; it was an accident. But if it had happened in the privacy of the massage room, instead of in a room full of people, his intentions may have been misconstrued.

Disrobing

Clients need to dress and undress in private, and they need to know that they do not have to undress at all if it makes them uncomfortable. Let them know that they can wear a bathing suit or whatever else is suitable—for instance, athletic shorts and a comfortable bra or tank top. If necessary, you can explain how it will limit your ability to work with them if they choose to leave clothes on, but always make sure they know that they will be covered except for whatever body part you will be working with at the time, that it is their decision, and avoid making them feel badly about it.

Locked Doors

The question of whether or not the door was locked has been a crucial point in some court cases in which a practitioner was sued for sexual harassment. Even if a client isn't locked in or could unlock the door, the point has been raised that the client should be able to leave the room quickly and easily. In many situations, a practitioner may want to lock the door to protect the client from unwanted intrusion, such as a stranger wandering into an office by mistake. A cautious way to handle that type of situation is to explain your reasons for wanting to lock the door and give clients the option of it being locked or unlocked. When there are multiple treatment rooms, it's easy to make a mistake and enter the wrong one; I've done it myself in my own office and unintentionally burst in on someone else's session.

Intrusive Work

Some manual therapies can involve intrusive work. If you have good reason to work in an area near a client's genitals, such as the attachments of thigh muscles, near the coccyx, or near a woman's breasts, you can tell the client in a matter-of-fact way what your intentions are and why it would help them. Use terms they can understand—breastbone or tailbone, for instance, instead of sternum or coccyx. Or if you use anatomical terms, make sure they understand where you will be working. "It might be a good idea to work on the muscles around your tailbone because it could be useful to free them up. However, if that makes you uncomfortable, it's fine to skip that area." Having a muscle chart in your room, or an anatomy app that you can show to clients is helpful. Let clients decide if it's all right. Watch to see if it really is okay, or whether they tense up or seem to be trying to act as if it's fine when it really isn't. The safest plan is to let clients know before the session begins that the session might involve intrusive work and get their consent before they are in the more vulnerable state of being on the table. In some jurisdictions, practitioners are required to get prior consent in writing for such work.

CONSIDER THIS

In my own state of North Carolina, massage therapists may perform massage in body cavities below the waist, which was not originally in our rules, but was successfully lobbied for by a medical massage association. It's presently a rare state of affairs, but those associations may successfully lobby other states for the right as time goes by. The rules governing body cavity massage are very strict. The client must have a written prescription or order from a licensed medical doctor for the treatment; the therapist must obtain specific written informed consent stating that work will be performed inside body cavities, and stating whether the client chooses to have a third party of their own choice in the room, or are giving permission to work with only the therapist in the room. As with all informed consent, the client has the right to withdraw that at any time, and should never be made to feel bad about doing so. Bear in mind at all times that internal work requires another whole level of diligence in adhering to professionalism and sensitivity.

Cautious behavior protects both you and your clients. In the altered state that clients enter into, they can get confused about both your intentions and where your hands actually are. Bring those things into their conscious awareness by giving clients specifics.

You may not know what areas are sensitive for a particular client, or what may bring up a particular memory for an abuse victim. If someone was pinned down by her shoulders during abuse, working in that area could bring up the memory, and yet, placing the hands on the anterior shoulders to help them relax toward the table is something that most therapists do in every session. We need to be conscious that any work has the potential to trigger a memory of sexual abuse; we don't have to be near the pelvis or breasts for an unpleasant association to arise. Therefore, you always want to keep an eye out for signs of discomfort from the client, such as their becoming more tense or reporting numbness.

Expressions of Affection

Although it may come from genuine caring, initiating hugs with clients isn't a good idea. Mandatory hugs can be very intrusive for clients. The same is true, only more so, for kissing on the forehead or cheek. We may think that clients would welcome any expressions of affection, but we may be wrong about that. As the client is leaving the session, you can show through your body language that you are available for a hug if the client wants to initiate one (assuming that you are open to it, and there's nothing wrong with you if you aren't) without forcing the issue. Giving clients the choice is another way to respect their boundaries. Again, we need to be aware of maintaining a professional demeanor, without appearing stuffy. If you don't want to hug a client and you think they're about to initiate it, you extend your hand to shake hands while smiling and saying "Thank you for coming, I'll see you at your next appointment."

Unintentional Touching

When asked about uncomfortable experiences, clients often cite situations in which some part of a practitioner's body other than hands touched them or the practitioner leaned against them. This is usually accidental on the part of the practitioner, but it can be disturbing to the client. One woman reports:

> ➤ *In the middle of a massage from a male practitioner, he leaned against my hip with his belly to reach the other side of me, instead of walking around the table. I was so uncomfortable that I had a difficult time relaxing for the rest of the session, wondering whether there would be another incident.*

Not every client will react strongly to unintentional or careless touching. However, some will. You do not want to prop yourself against clients as if they were furniture. Of course, if your technique requires you to touch clients with other parts of your body or to lean against them, the reasons for this intrusiveness should be explained to clients, and their consent must be given.

You also want to be careful about wearing sleeves that dangle and things that could brush against clients. Therapists with longer hair should wear a ponytail or other style to make certain that their hair never touches the client as they're bending over the body. In the open and receptive state induced by bodywork, clients shouldn't have to figure out what is touching them.

The Power of Touch

We cannot ignore sexual issues when learning to work with our clients. Because the sensuality of the tender, healing touch that we offer is often so close to the sensuality of sex, we need to be all the more careful to maintain clear sexual boundaries with clients. The manual therapies are intimate and can bring up issues about sexuality, both for us and for our clients. We are touching unclothed bodies, which many people have only experienced in the context of sex.

This work can be a blessing for people who are starved for safe and respectful touch. However, we're always skirting the edge between the sacred and the profane. It speaks to the goodwill and compassion of practitioners that we so often succeed in keeping the balance on the side of the sacred.

Questions for Reflection

1. Has a manual therapy practitioner or other health-care provider ever said or done something that felt like a violation of your sexual boundaries or that made you uncomfortable? Did you say something to the practitioner, either at the time or later? Did you tell anyone? If this has not happened to you, have you heard of such an incident happening to a friend or colleague? What feelings did that person have about the incident?

2. Have you ever looked up to or had a crush on a practitioner of any kind who worked closely with you? Do you feel that it would have been appropriate if the practitioner had entered into a romantic relationship with you? Why or why not?

3. Is there anything in your history that might help you be more sensitive to issues of sexual boundaries with clients? Is there anything that might get in the way of your being comfortable with setting clear sexual boundaries with clients?

4. Imagine that you're single and run into an ex-client (also single) at a party. There seems to be a mutual attraction that you weren't aware of while you were working with the client. You are thinking of asking this person for a date. As a professional, what concerns would you have in evaluating whether it would be ethical or wise to do so?

5. Have you ever had a professional massage in which the draping wasn't adequate? Were you uncomfortable because of it? If you weren't, could you imagine circumstances in which you would be?

thePoint To learn more about the concepts discussed in this chapter, visit http://thePoint .lww.com/Allen-McIntosh4e

CHAPTER 8

Sexual Boundaries: Protecting Ourselves

We live in a culture in which massage is sometimes associated with sex. Many people are uneducated about the manual therapies and do not appreciate that we are trained professionals who work with therapeutic intention. It's distressing but understandable that some of the public might still think that all massage practitioners offer sexual services. How often have we seen massage therapists portrayed in television sitcoms or movies as crossing the line? How often have new acquaintances made sexual innuendoes and jokes about our work? When traveling, I've personally

The intimacy of our work leaves us open to misunderstandings and false accusations.

noticed billboard advertising that is truly blatant. There's one advertisement for a "spa" about two hours away from my home that actually has a silhouette of a naked woman on it. I recently saw another one that stated, "Open 24 Hours! Truckers welcome!" No wonder the public still gets that impression of massage. To complicate matters, those who do offer sexual services often bill themselves as practicing massage, since there are only a couple of places in the United

States where prostitution itself is legal. Sex workers can't honestly advertise what they do, so they fall back on using massage as a front for it.

Protecting Yourself from the Public's Misunderstanding

Unfortunately, the accusations aren't always false. Somatic practitioners do sometimes cross ethical boundaries about sexual behavior—probably no more than other professionals do, but our profession is particularly vulnerable to being linked with sex. When other practitioners violate sexual boundaries, it can damage not only their own reputations but also those of the ethical professionals in their community. How do we protect ourselves from potential confusion and harm, both from the public and from within our ranks?

Mistaken Identity

Whether you are in private practice or work in a spa or even a medical office, you may not be able to avoid the occasional low moment of someone assuming that you are offering sexual services, or testing the water to see what sort of reaction they get from you. If you have your own practice and advertise publicly, you have to be prepared for the occasional inappropriate or offensive questions on the phone. Here's an example:

> ➤ *A colleague was befuddled when a prospective client asked if she provided "a happy ending." Not having heard this euphemism for sexual release, she said, "Oh, yes, I like my clients to enjoy their massages." When he then described what he wanted in plainer language, she was quick to tell him she didn't offer sexual services and that she wouldn't work with him if that was what he wanted.*

While fielding such questions on the phone can be uncomfortable, dealing in person with a client who expects sex can be annoying and frightening. Although it's only a remote possibility, this situation could also be dangerous, especially if you work alone.

Self-Protection: Working for Others

While those in private practice are more vulnerable, those who work for someone else also need to be careful in choosing their employers. If you are employed, you want to make sure in the initial interview that your employer has strict policies banning sexually inappropriate behavior by clients and that those policies are made known to all clients. Select an employer you know will back you up if you choose to end a session or choose not to work with a client who has made sexual innuendos or requests.

It's an unfortunate fact that some employers are not sympathetic to practitioners, and just expect them to deal with it without any management support. They don't want to lose business, even that of someone who acts inappropriately.

Self-Protection: Private Practice

There may be no foolproof way to avoid clients who are sexually inappropriate, but there are ways you can lessen their frequency and protect yourself.

Choose Your Clients Well

Those in private practice need to take care in choosing their clients. Those who do outcalls and those who practice at home, or in an office where they are alone, should be extra careful. Some female practitioners avoid these problems altogether

I was working in a chiropractic office owned by two chiropractors. Several therapists worked there, and the chiropractors just ignored any complaints from us about sexual behavior. One day I was giving a man a massage, and he made the comment that I had a beautiful body and asked if I would do a house call. I stopped and told him I was a professional therapist and that I do not do anything sexual, and I would appreciate it if he refrained from further comments. He said okay, but a few minutes later, I could see his erection waving around under the sheet. I asked him to turn over, and as soon as he did, he started grinding himself on the table. We weren't allowed to have our own music playing in the treatment rooms; they had music that was piped through the whole building, and at that moment, Marvin Gaye came over the speakers singing "Sexual Healing." If the situation wasn't so pathetic, it would have been funny. I just took my hands off him, told him the massage was over and to get dressed, grabbed my purse, and told the chiropractor on my way out the door that I quit.

—K.M., LMT

by limiting their practice to female clients. (Women clients are generally less sexually aggressive than men. They can be seductive, for instance, but aren't as likely either to expect sexual services or to ask for them.) Some practitioners don't work with anyone who hasn't been referred by someone they trust.

Advertising and Business Cards

Regardless of your gender, if you advertise or post your business card in a public place, you may attract the wrong kind of client. Be careful when you advertise in a publication. Find out where your ad will be placed. Will it run next to the ads in which "massage" is a code word for sex? Will it show up next to ads for places with dubious names such as Buffy's Massage and Pleasure Spa? If so, you might want to reconsider advertising in that publication. A lot of businesses and public places have bulletin boards on their premises. While you might post a business card on the bulletin board at your local library or local community college, you might not want to post one in a bar.

It's also helpful to consider the nature of a publication's readership. If you live in a big city, running an ad in a smaller, weekly, more trendy newspaper is usually safer than using the classifieds in the daily newspaper or Craigslist. Readers of the smaller papers are often more attuned to alternative health practices; it's a good idea to obtain several back issues and check out the advertisements before you decide to advertise. Wherever you advertise, it's also a good idea to avoid the words "release," "total relaxation," and "full-body massage." These phrases can sound like veiled sexual references. Avoid them too when you're on the phone with prospective clients.

Make sure your business card doesn't send a mixed message. Cards that give no last name, that simply say "Massage by Bill" or "Relaxing Massage by Jennifer," are less professional and may give clients the impression you have something to hide. Since sex workers usually don't give their last names when they advertise, it's important that you provide your full name and credentials, such as professional association membership, state license number (which is required in most regulated states on any advertising), and so forth to establish that you're a legitimate massage therapist. Using the term "therapeutic massage" and naming your particular specialty, such as sports massage, are also helpful. To ensure your privacy and professionalism, list your business number, not your personal one when possible. Many therapists operate with only a cell phone these days, and don't have a number that is specifically dedicated to business. If that is the case, it's wise to make your voice mail message professional, anyway. Your friends and family will know you're using the same phone for business and personal calls, so leave a message such as "You've reached Laura Allen, Licensed Massage Therapist. Please leave your name and number and I'll return your call."

A quick search on the Internet will reveal that people offering sexual massage often have websites that make it pretty clear what they're doing, although they may not actually say they're offering sex. A picture of the "therapist" wearing lingerie is a pretty good clue!

Screening Clients by Phone

Clients who are looking for more than just a massage may not always say so in the initial phone call. Before the prevalence of cell phones, it was easier to figure out which prospective clients wanted something else. When I first started out as a massage therapist, there was a type of call that I called "the dreaded phone booth call." When I could hear traffic in the background, I always said I wasn't in. The traffic noise told me that these people were calling from a phone booth, and it seemed too likely that the callers were avoiding calling from their home or office because they thought they were doing something illicit.

Since almost everyone uses cell phones these days, the sound of traffic noise is not unusual anymore; however, there are other red flags that signal the wrong kind of call. If people call on Friday afternoon around 5 p.m., they may be more likely to be facing a weekend alone and looking for "companionship." Such callers often don't want to make an appointment unless you can see them immediately, within an hour or two. Also, look out for callers who initially don't give their full name or who give no name at all.

While the majority of us prefer the term "massage therapist," I have visited places where there is no stigma at all attached to the terms "masseur" and "masseuse." In fact, online dictionaries define those terms as "one who gives professional massage," "one who practices massage and physiotherapy," and so forth, and has no sexual references.

Here are some other ways to screen out clients who are calling for the wrong reason:

Ask for Information

Ask for callers' full names and callback numbers. If they refuse, don't make the appointment. Also, you can ask about their previous experience with massage. If they've been to a massage therapist you know is legitimate or if they seem to be familiar with professional bodywork, that's a good sign.

Clarify Your Boundaries

When in doubt, you can say, "I like to make it clear to all new clients that I offer only a nonsexual, therapeutic massage." This is not always convincing, however, because sex workers who call themselves masseuses or masseurs will say the same thing in case the caller is from the vice squad.

Trust Your Intuition

If you have an uneasy feeling about someone, don't make the appointment.

If you have an uneasy feeling about someone, don't make the appointment. It is better to lose a session fee than to put yourself in danger. You may always say you are fully booked, or you are not currently accepting new clients.

Staying Safe during the Session

Usually, the worst a client interested in sexual services does is injure your professional dignity and pride. However, in rare cases, massage therapists have been assaulted by such clients. As long as there's even a slight danger, there's no need to take risks. Here are some ways to stay safe:

Work in a Safe Setting

Working in an office building is usually safer and appears more professional to prospective clients than working out of your home. Leading a client through your home to where the bedrooms are (and your office now is) can be suggestive to new clients.

Massage therapists, especially those who are just starting out and working alone, are faced with striking a balance between trying to build their business, and keeping their own safety in mind. While you may not want to turn down business, you're always taking a chance if you work alone in an isolated office or home with clients you don't know. If you choose to work alone, it's best to choose office space in a location where other businesses or professional offices are around. A few safety measures that can be taken:

- Avoid scheduling new clients late in the day when someone with sexual intentions might assume that no one else will be coming in.
- Keep your car key and your phone (volume off, of course) on your person in case you feel threatened and need to make a quick escape. Nothing in your office (or in someone's home, as mentioned later about outcalls) is worth your safety. Leave it and you can come back with another person (the police, if there was any actual inappropriate touching on the part of the client or grabbing you involved—that's considered assault) in tow.
- Remember that an intake interview not only serves the purpose of gathering pertinent information about the client, it serves for client and therapist to establish rapport. If someone makes you suspicious about their intentions during the intake interview, reiterate to them that you only practice therapeutic massage; remember that we have the right of refusal as well as the client, and you don't have to let them on the table.

Be Especially Careful About Outcalls

Outcalls require you to go into someone else's home, office, hotel room or other location, and be at the mercy of any hidden agendas the client might have. Screen such calls carefully or do outcalls only with people who have been referred by someone you trust.

➤ *One male massage therapist related a story of being set up by a female client who wanted to make her boyfriend jealous. During the outcall, the client threw the draping off her chest just as her boyfriend burst through the door. The boyfriend made angry accusations and the massage therapist fled, unharmed but wiser.*

When going on an outcall, call a friend or family member when you arrive. Let them know the address where you are, and what time you will check back in with them. Always have someone who can check on you if they don't hear from you by a certain time, even if you have to pay for the service. Answering services will often provide such a service as reminder calls. If you are doing outcalls in a hotel, stop at the front desk and tell them what room you are going to and when you should be down.

Spell Out Your Policies in Writing

As part of their intake process, some massage therapists ask new clients to sign an agreement stating that the practitioner has the right to terminate a session if the client speaks or acts inappropriately. The clearer you can make it from the beginning that this is a nonsexual massage, the easier it will be for you to avoid inappropriate requests.

Educating Clients: Setting Limits

No matter whether you are in private practice or work for an employer, you need to know how to set limits with a client who asks for sexual services. There is no set way to respond when a client on the table asks you for something that is inappropriate. It depends on your own comfort level, how safe the setting is, and your history with the client. When a client misunderstands what you are offering, you don't need to waste your energy on a fit of righteous indignation. Some clients are simply misinformed; sometimes all you have to do is educate them and set clear limits.

If a client makes an inappropriate sexual suggestion during the session, respond to it immediately. Hesitating will give the client the impression that you may be open to the idea.

- Stop the massage.
- Take your hands off the client's body and take a step back from the table.
- Address the situation.
- Define your boundaries.

You can say, "I want to make it clear that this is a nonsexual massage, and I won't work with anyone who is acting inappropriately." Others, depending on their comfort level, might give a client who has made an inappropriate remark a chance to improve his or her behavior. Sometimes a client doesn't intend to be offensive; he or she just doesn't know better. Of course, if the client is being obviously aggressive—physically stimulating him- or herself or trying to grab you—then you should end the massage, letting him or her know you are stepping out of the room and that you expect the person to put on his or her clothes and leave. (With such a client, you would want to enlist someone else to wait with you, if possible.)

Also, if you're not sure what the client's intentions are but still feel uncomfortable or threatened by their comments or behavior, trust your feelings and end the session. You can say, "Perhaps you don't mean any harm, but I'm not comfortable working with you anymore. I'll wait outside while you get dressed."

Most massage therapists are so grateful when these clients leave that they don't ask for payment. (Others get payment at the start of a session.) Technically, clients may owe the fee for a massage or half a massage, but it's up to you whether to make an issue of it. Of course, if you work for someone else, you need to know their policies about such a situation.

Boundary Lessons

It was stressed in my class in massage school to acknowledge any sexual overtures immediately, whether it's a comment or anything else inappropriate. I was nervous the first time it happened to me, but I remembered the lesson: if you don't address it immediately, you have just given the client permission to carry on with whatever inappropriate behavior he or she was committing. In spite of all efforts to exhibit professional behavior, there are still people who will test your boundaries. It doesn't happen often, but when it does, I always remember that lesson and speak up right then to let them know it won't be tolerated. One warning, and then they're out.

—J.E., LMT

Self-Presentation

If you're getting a high percentage of calls or office encounters in which the clients think you're offering sex, you need to take a look at how you're presenting yourself. This could be as simple as changing your ads or how you dress or as complicated as looking at what your intentions really are. You might need to get another perspective—you could ask a mentor or more experienced practitioner for honest feedback.

This has become much more of an issue since social media became popular. If you identify yourself as a massage therapist on your social media, beware of the image you're putting out there. If you're casual about your privacy settings, you should assume that anyone in the world may see the pictures of you lounging by the pool in a barely-there bikini and a pina colada in hand. There are plenty of people who troll the Internet just looking for opportunities.

Perhaps the day will come that when people think of massage, they think only of its many health benefits and the boost it gives to both physical and emotional well-being. Until that time, clear communication in all stages of our contacts with clients can help educate those who need it and protect us from misunderstandings.

The Erection Dilemma: Protecting Both Ourselves and Our Clients

How should a practitioner respond when a client has an erection during the session? Again, it depends on the situation, the client, and your comfort level. Some practitioners wrongly believe that if a man is having an erection, the practitioner must immediately end the massage. There is the misconception that for a man to have an erection, he must be deliberately sexualizing the situation and either mentally or physically stimulating himself. However, the truth is that having an erection can be an innocent accident and just as embarrassing to the client as it may be anxiety-producing for the practitioner.

If a client gets an erection and doesn't acknowledge it at all or say or do anything inappropriate, or if he acknowledges it in embarrassment, or if he is sleepy and relaxed at the time, there's no need to get upset over that. Be cautious about jumping to the wrong conclusion and accusing someone of sexual behavior just because an erection occurs.

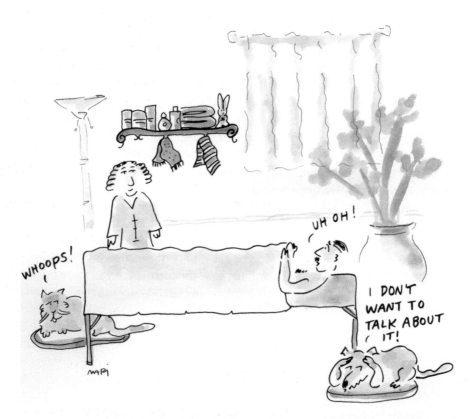

Erections can occur as a natural physiological response to being touched. One of my teachers in massage school described them as being like "a dog wagging his tail"—an automatic physiological response to pleasure. Men report that they can be floating along enjoying the sensuality of a massage without any sexual thoughts or feelings of attraction to the therapist, and then . . . oops, their enjoyment has become visible. Younger men can have erections, as one therapist put it, "if the wind changes direction," and certainly from the intimacy of a massage.

When an erection occurs, it can make both the client and the practitioner feel vulnerable. If you respond with unnecessary disapproval and fear, it's a disservice to an already embarrassed client. Yet you have to guard against the threat of a disrespectful, abusive client. It's a tricky situation.

Aside from the misconception that a man is in total control over whether he has an erection and that any erection that happens during a session is deliberately caused, there are other common areas of confusion.

Sometimes bodyworkers assume that if a client doesn't say anything or look uncomfortable, having an erection does not bother him. However, many men say that at such a time, they are embarrassed but decide to keep quiet, hoping the therapist won't notice. You have to remember that even the possibility of having an erection keeps many men from seeking a professional massage.

Sometimes practitioners think that if a client is aroused or has made sexual remarks or requests, they (the practitioners) have done something wrong to cause the arousal or that they have somehow given the client a mixed message. Massage therapists can feel a sense of shame at such times, as if they have been encouraging the client in some way. That confusion can make practitioners uncertain about how to respond. Especially, if you don't know the client well, the situation can be uncomfortable, awkward, and even scary. Most massage therapists report that it's rare in their practice for a man to have an erection. If clients (of either sex) are frequently aroused by your work, you want to figure out if you are somehow sending out sexual signals.

Your goal is to protect yourself, your dignity, and your reputation without humiliating a client who means no harm.

First, make an assessment. Is this a natural physiological response, or is the client deliberately arousing himself? What has been your history with this client? If you have no reason to mistrust a client—for instance, you've worked with the client many times before and he's never tried to cross sexual territory—you might continue working and assume that his response is innocent. However, if this is a new client who has already given you reason to mistrust him or a client who has

---

REAL EXPERIENCE

My wife and I attended massage school together. One day while we were still students, I was giving her a massage, and she calmly said "Your penis is on my arm." I stepped back and said "What??" She said, "It's okay, it's *me*, but you weren't even aware of it. The way you were leaning over me, your crotch was right on my arm." She was right—I wasn't even aware of it—I was focused on the massage. I started right then making an effort to be totally conscious about my own body mechanics when doing massage. A client could easily misinterpret your intentions if you're not careful!

—C.A., LMBT

skirted the edges of decency before, then your choices will be different. Or if you're not sure what the client's intentions are, then you have another course of action.

Clients Who Are Having a Natural, Unintentional Response

What should you do when you notice that your client has an erection and you're pretty certain that it is just a physiological response? Should you ignore it or say something? And if you say something, what should you say and when should you say it? Is it a good idea to talk with new male clients about the possibility that they could have an erection? All of that depends on the client's behavior, your professional relationship with the client, and your assessment of him. Depending on all that, you have these choices:

Ignore It

Under the theory that what goes up must come down, practitioners often choose to ignore an erection. If the client isn't acting inappropriately, most bodyworkers probably wouldn't interrupt the flow of a massage unless the client says something.

Work on a More Neutral Part of the Body

You can keep doing what you're doing, move to a less intimate part of the body, or ask the client to turn over. Or if you know, for instance, that working on his abdomen or thighs gets a client stirred up, you can work with that area earlier in the massage when he's less relaxed. You also have the option of totally avoiding an area the client finds stimulating. However, you don't want to make a practice of limiting the range of your massage simply because of your personal discomfort.

Clear the Air: Say Something

It's not unusual for practitioners, especially women, to be uncomfortable about dealing with a client having an erection. While men and women practitioners seem to feel equally violated by a client who expects sex and is being offensive, men seem to have more locker-room ease with a client who has an unintentional erection.

Regardless of your gender, if you think that silence might be adding to your discomfort or the client's, then it's a good idea to clear the air. You can say something such as, "It's natural to have an unintentional physical response to massage." If you think he's embarrassed or he says he is, you can say something such as, "Oh, that happens sometimes. Would you be more comfortable if you turned over?" or "Try focusing on your breathing." Speak in a matter-of-fact way and without disapproval. While some suggest that you place a towel over the groin, most think that would only draw attention to the area without communicating a clear message.

Clients Who Are Questionable or Over the Line

If you're either not sure of the client's intentions or pretty sure that they are out of bounds, use the same tactics as for responding to a client who is sexualizing the situation: Stop the massage and define your boundaries with a statement such as, "I want to be sure that you know that this is a nonsexual massage. I will end the session if you are looking for something else."

Depending on the response or on your comfort level or your intuition, either state that the massage is over or proceed with caution, letting them know that you will end the massage if they continue being offensive.

Education before the Session

Whether to say something before a session begins is a judgment call made on a case-by-case basis. For instance, it might be helpful to talk with a client if he usually gets erections during the massage. Talk with him before he has taken off his clothes or gotten on the table. You could say, "I noticed you had an erection during the last massage, and I wanted to clear the air and say that I know that erections are usually just a physiological response to touch and it's not unusual for clients to have them." If he is a relatively new client, you could add, "Since you're a new client, I want to make it clear that this isn't a sexual massage." A legitimate client shouldn't be offended and might be relieved.

Of course, if a client expresses concern before the massage about having an erection, then you want to educate him that erections can happen without sexual intent and they aren't necessarily a cause for concern. A colleague had a humorous way to clarify the boundaries for an elderly client with a twinkle in his eye who asked, "What if I get an erection?" She said, "If you don't pay any attention to it, I won't, either." I once personally had an elderly client who signed the section on the intake form relating to inappropriate comments or behavior, and he said "You don't have to worry about me. I've got ED (erectile dysfunction)!"

Most massage therapists say they don't bring up the possibility of an erection unless the client mentions it. They think that even saying "You might have an erection" could make a client wonder if you're sexualizing the situation. Of course, that's not always the case. For instance, if a white-haired grandmotherly massage therapist talked to an 18-year-old man about what's normal, he would probably appreciate the reassurance.

Support and Suggestions

If you still find yourself anxious about a client having an erection even though you know it's an innocent response, you could talk with colleagues and mentors for support and advice. Unless you limit your practice to women, you will occasionally encounter erections.

This work is intimate, and nowhere is that more evident than with "the erection dilemma." The potential embarrassments on both sides challenge us to hone our communication and boundary-setting skills. Whether we're dealing with a major creep or a minor "oops," we're called on to use our professional judgment and our common sense. It's all just part of the job.

Protecting Ourselves from Ethics Complaints or Legal Charges

Chapter 5 discusses keeping good framework and boundaries as a way to avoid ethics complaints. This section focuses specifically on ethical issues related to sexual complaints. Although maintaining good boundaries and solid framework is always a protection against ethics complaints, some red flags and troublesome situations are unique to sexual issues.

Here are some warnings that may help you make your way through the troublesome situations that can arise:

No One is Immune

Any practitioner can be complained against by any client. Any practitioner, male or female, gay or straight, can be accused of sexually violating a client. Seductive or careless practitioners are not the only ones accused. Even good-hearted, conscientious practitioners can have clients misread their intentions.

Sexual abuse and violation issues are about power, and they cross all lines of gender and sexual orientation.

Practitioners can be accused by clients of the same sex, for instance, as the case below shows. Sexual abuse and violation issues are about power, and they cross all lines of gender and sexual orientation.

The body holds the unconscious, and the unconscious is often primitive and irrational. That's why we have to provide clear boundaries when we do this work.

➤ *A heterosexual female practitioner was working around a female client's sacrum and was suddenly accused by the client of violating her anally. The practitioner was horrified and immediately removed her hands from the client. She worked the rest of the session to calm the client's concerns, but the client never seemed to regain trust in her and stopped coming for sessions.*

In retrospect, the practitioner realized she might have avoided the misunderstanding if she'd taken more care. There are a number of ways she most likely could have avoided the misunderstanding: (1) by asking the client to leave on her underwear or by working on top of the draping, (2) by getting the informed consent of the client (during the session she could have explained where she wanted to work and the purpose of working in that area and then asked the client's permission), or (3) by postponing the work. If she thought the client was too deep into an altered state to give informed consent at that point, she could have not worked in that area for that session. Then, at the next session, before the client was on the table, she could explain the possible need to work in that area and ask for the client's consent.

CONSIDER THIS

It should never be assumed that only male clients make sexual overtures to massage therapists. Many male therapists have reported being flirted with and openly propositioned by clients; it's happened to the male therapists who have worked in my own office. The burden is on us all, no matter or our gender or sexual orientation, to keep our own sexual desires out of the massage room. If you're a therapist who has been lonely and seeking a relationship or missing sex, for example, the thought of "Why not?" when propositioned by someone may pop into your head. Banish that immediately. A few minutes of fun and/or gratification is not worth the possible consequences of loss of reputation, loss of license, or worse, should the word get out.

No one is immune to being misunderstood by a client. However, if you consistently attend to framework and boundaries, you'll be more likely to head off trouble from the start.

Some Are at Greater Risk

Although anyone can be complained against, if you are in a group that is generally perceived as sexually aggressive, whether or not that perception is accurate, you may be more likely to be complained about or sued. Since most complaints are by female clients against male practitioners, men, as a whole, are more at risk. In conservative parts of the country, minority men can be even further at risk, as can homosexual practitioners. All of us who touch people need to be cautious about sexual boundaries, but practitioners in those groups should be extra careful.

Seductive Clients Call for Proper Boundaries

There are instances of seductive clients causing problems for male bodyworkers. The situation could arise between a client and a practitioner of opposite genders or between a client and a practitioner of the same gender.

CONSIDER THIS

After licensing was implemented in my state, males practitioners were accused the very first year. Our board was in existence for 10 years before a male accused a female therapist of sexual impropriety. In reality, there were probably more instances where it happened, but men are much less likely to come forward to complain about a woman doing something inappropriate.

➤ *A male massage school teacher allowed a female client, who had recently been a student in his class, to seduce him. He described that she had "an exquisite sense" of how to connect with him and make him feel special. He said, "She made me feel that making love to her was a heroic and generous act." But her unbalanced nature soon showed when she began to talk publicly about their sexual relationship as though she had been an unwilling victim. Her stories damaged the teacher's reputation.*

In this instance, the practitioner did violate his client's sexual boundaries; it was unethical to have sex with a client and further poor judgment to have a sexual relationship with a recent student, but even practitioners who don't violate any boundaries can be falsely accused.

➤ *A male bodyworker described narrowly escaping a disaster when a client pleaded with him to have sex with her. She gave him assurances that she wasn't the type to get attached. When he still refused, she retaliated: She went to the police to check the legalities of his license, and she called his landlord and reported he was having wild orgies. None of these actions caused him permanent damage, but he was glad that he had been firm in his refusal.*

How do you guard against such emotionally-disturbed clients? What are the warning signs? Sometimes you can tell by the feelings these clients bring up in you. One red flag is feeling the need to rescue the client. The bodyworkers in these stories reported feeling that they were, as one put it, "nobly responding to the true needs of the client" by becoming intimate. He said, "I thought of my client as an extraordinarily sensitive being who only needed support and recognition to realize her full potential."

When you feel like a noble rescuer, you may be responding to the client's deep need to be saved. This kind of intense transference from a client is highly volatile and can, as the stories show, quickly change to disappointment and rage.

Another warning sign is a feeling of specialness—that either the client or you are special and do not have to stay within normal boundaries. Some mentally unbalanced clients are experts at making practitioners feel special. They know just the right buttons to push.

The intensity of the feelings of specialness goes beyond normal transference. If a client makes you feel unusually attractive, competent, or sensitive and is suggesting that the two of you become lovers, or if you have started thinking about that possibility, you are in a dangerous situation.

Your countertransference in these cases can feel as if a spell has been cast over you. You can break the spell by getting a good dose of reality from a grounded

REAL EXPERIENCE

I had an appointment with a new female client. She was a voluptuous woman, attractive and personable, and gave no clue while we were in the lobby that she was seeking anything other than therapeutic massage. She stated during the intake that her back bothered her a lot.

I escorted her to the treatment room and left her to get undressed, telling her I would start the massage face up. I had just begun the massage, and had my hands on her head, when she pulled the cover down and exposed her very large breasts. She put her hands on them and pushed them up and said, "Carrying this load around is why my back hurts!" I was shocked, but I quickly recovered, stood up so I could look her in the eye, and pulled the draping up over her. I said "Ma'am, draping is required here and I will have to ask you not to expose yourself again." She apologized, and I carried on with the massage. I don't know what kind of reaction she was expecting, but I don't think that was it.

—W.C., CMT

professional you trust. And you can also remember this: There's never a good reason to have sex with a client or student or even a recent ex-client or ex-student, and in nearly every regulated state, it's against the law for a specified period of time.

Getting a consultation from a trained mental health professional can help you understand the dynamics of the situation. Seductive clients, for instance, do not always want you to be their lover; they're telling you how they habitually deal with power in relationships. They're telling you how they usually get into trouble in their lives or how they get attention. A consultant can help you protect yourself and the client by not playing into the client's unhealthy patterns.

Be Aware of the "Nice Guy" Blind Spot

As well as being aware of clients who may play on our vulnerabilities, we have to be aware of our own blind spots. Many of us don't fully appreciate all the effects of transference; however, the danger is greater for male practitioners who don't have a good enough grasp of this dynamic. If these practitioners don't fully realize the power of women's unconscious attitudes about men and the possible memories of sexual abuse that women may bring to the table, they can be stepping into trouble. Some men may think that because they are "nice guys" or happily married, female clients will somehow automatically feel comfortable with them, which is simply not true.

Similarly, the take-charge behavior that is expected of men in many situations may not serve them well as manual therapists. Here's an example:

> *A male massage therapy student was partnered with a female student to learn the techniques for back work. When he began working, he unsnapped her bra without asking her. A teacher noticed both what he'd done and the woman's startled reaction. When the male student was asked to explain his actions, he said, "I thought it would be easier for me to get to her back muscles without the bra in the way." He didn't have any inappropriate intent, but it was a thoughtless action, and the client doesn't realize that without clear communication. The next time the situation occurred, he remembered to ask permission.*

It's understandable for a student to be focused on learning technique, but goal-oriented behavior isn't necessarily helpful in manual therapists. As practitioners, men are safer from misunderstandings if they let the client run the show. Clients need to know they are in charge of what happens, especially when the gender dynamics involve a male practitioner and a female client. In this case, for example, the student should have asked permission to unhook the woman's bra, explaining the therapeutic reason for it. We can note that many female students—and therapists—have done the same thing with no ill intentions, but it's still a violation of the client's boundaries.

It's not fair, but it's a fact, that male massage therapists have their own set of problems to contend with. That may be why about 80% of therapists are female. There are a certain amount of females who don't feel comfortable with a male therapist, and that's not always related to any past issues of sexual abuse. Sometimes it may be a body image issue, or just plain modesty in front of members of the opposite sex. Then there are women who wouldn't mind at all getting a massage from a male, but their spouse objects to it because they have the "I don't want another man putting their hands on my woman" mentality. And then there are homophobic males who don't want another male touching them in an intimate manner. While female therapists may have to deal with the occasional sexual overture, male therapists come to the table with ready-made obstacles through no fault of their own.

We want to *all* be especially careful to guard against the kind of behavior that could be misunderstood or that could cause us trouble, either the relatively minor trouble of losing a client, or the major trouble of a complaint filed against us with the massage board, a lawsuit, or even an accusation of sexual assault resulting in an arrest.

Protecting the Profession

There are people in every profession who use their roles to take advantage of clients sexually, and ours is no exception. To protect the profession, we need to distinguish between the well-intentioned practitioner who stumbles into a destructive situation or makes a mistake in judgment and the practitioner who habitually seduces clients or violates their sexual boundaries and who is indifferent to the emotional damage he causes. This practitioner is considered a predator and is the most damaging to clients and the reputation of the profession. Unfortunately, there are some predators out there who figure the massage profession would be a good environment to meet new victims.

Predatory Behavior

Predators are practitioners who deliberately misuse the power of transference to take advantage of their clients sexually. They may date clients, misusing the affection and attachment that some clients feel toward them. Or they may be sexually inappropriate during a session—taking advantage of the client's trust, altered state, and reluctance to question their actions.

Predators who cross boundaries during a session generally follow a pattern. They start by being friendly and gaining the client's trust, then during the session, they "accidentally" touch the client's genitals or a woman's breast. If the client says nothing, the practitioner continues, gradually touching the client with more sexual intent. Clients often report feeling confused by this but fear they will insult the therapist if they question him. To add to the confusion, sometimes the practitioner has been referred by the client's friends, who spoke well of him. Clients may find it hard to believe the "friendly" practitioner is doing something inappropriate. In some instances, a client's confusion and passivity are related to a history of sexual abuse. This experience can be psychologically harmful to any client, but especially those who have suffered childhood abuse.

In other cases, the client participates, flirting with the practitioner and even consenting to sexual behavior. However, even if the client has appeared to give consent, the practitioner has committed a serious breach of ethics. The responsibility of ethical professional behavior is not on the client—it's on us.

The responsibility of ethical professional behavior is not on the client—it's on us.

Over the years, our profession has become increasingly sensitive to sexual harassment and misuse of power. We have become increasingly aware of the damage that can be done by crossing these boundaries. We have come to understand that seductiveness isn't about sex and affection; it's about dominance and aggression. Practitioners involved in habitual predatory behavior are often sociopaths who have no concern about the harm done to others.

Later, when not in an altered state or in the presence of the engaging predator, victimized clients often begin to question the practitioner's actions. However, even when they realize they have been violated, they may be reluctant to make a complaint against the practitioner, not realizing that they are not the first and won't be the last to be mistreated by the predator. Also, they may find it hard to explain why they didn't protest at the time. Like many victims of sexual assault, they may not even want to tell a friend or family member, much less go to the police or massage board, in fear that it will become a public matter. Feeling violated seems twice as bad when the victim has to be publicly exposed.

No Witch Hunts

Habitual predators do great harm to clients and to the reputation of the profession. It's in the interest of the profession to find ways to expose them and shut them down. However, I'm not advocating witch hunts. You don't want to be quick to point the finger, jump into lawsuits, or drag people's names through the mud for little or no reason. There's no healing in such actions.

Be very careful about making accusations. Spreading rumors and unsubstantiated gossip can harm the reputation of an innocent person, affecting that person's livelihood. Aside from being unkind and unethical, it can make you vulnerable to slander suits from the accused. If a person has actually been arrested, tried, and convicted, or had his or her license taken away, that is a matter of public record. Until that point in time, it is gossip/hearsay and harmful to his or her reputation. From my time on our state board sitting in on disciplinary hearings, I can truthfully state that not every person who gets accused is guilty.

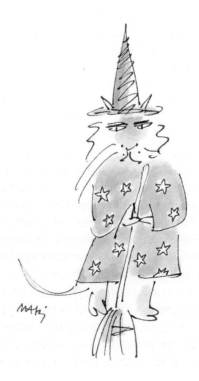

Dealing with Rumors of Sexual Misbehavior

As noted before, there are generally two different kinds of practitioners who are sexually inappropriate with clients: the well-intentioned practitioner who is momentarily off-balance and has made a bad judgment and the uncaring, habitual predator. It's important that colleagues, licensing boards, and boards of ethics recognize the difference and not be unnecessarily harsh with the well-meaning practitioner or too easy on the predator.

The main way you tell these two kinds of practitioners apart is by their histories and reputations. Even if a predator is recently graduated, he will often have been inappropriate in school. Another way to distinguish them is by how they react to being confronted. Approached in a diplomatic way, a well-meaning practitioner will usually be reasonable and even repentant, whereas predators may not return calls and, if they do, will become angry and vengeful.

Only the victimized clients themselves can file complaints with a licensing or ethics board or with the police. However, other practitioners may become involved out of concern for the reputation of the practitioner or the reputation of the profession. They may want to talk with the practitioner or provide emotional support or advice for clients who are lodging complaints.

There is the caveat that sometimes, predators may get away with their behavior for a long time with no accusations and no loss of reputation. Just like many rapes go unreported to law enforcement because of shame or fear that the victim is carrying around, some people who are assaulted by their massage therapist don't come forward, either. Sometimes, seeing that another person has come forward with a complaint results in others doing the same.

I was once asked to be an expert witness in the trial of a male therapist accused by a woman of sexually assaulting her. At the first trial, the accused person had about a half-dozen long-standing clients, most of them women, show up to be character witnesses for him. The proceedings had just started when the prosecutor asked for a continuance because he had received other complaints accusing the man, who had been practicing for many years. When the second trial was convened, the accused man's defense attorney came into the hallway within minutes and advised him to accept a plea bargain, because the prosecutor had produced 10 more women who claimed they had also been assaulted by the therapist. In another instance, after the license of a therapist was taken at a disciplinary hearing, the board received numerous letters from women saying things along the line of "Thank God this man was finally punished. He assaulted me years ago." If no one comes forward, then the predator may carry on unchecked for years.

If a client tells you that another therapist assaulted him or her, gently encourage the person to come forward and file a complaint, even if it happened years ago. It's not our job to add to someone's feelings of guilt, shame, or embarrassment, but a gentle reminder that if no one complains, the person is still out there preying on others might be the encouragement they need to come forward.

Dealing with a Practitioner Who Is Momentarily Off-Balance

Many practitioners, hearing rumors of a practitioner crossing the line with a client, will choose to ignore it; that's a better response than spreading a story you don't know to be true.

However, if you know the practitioner well enough to be concerned and you believe he or she is usually ethical, you may wish to contact him or her. You can approach the practitioner directly in a manner that shows you haven't yet drawn conclusions. Perhaps you could call or write to the person: "I've heard this about you. I thought you needed to know what is being said so that you can respond to it." While the practitioner may be defensive, many in those circumstances would appreciate hearing the rumors. Unless there is a client who wants your support in filing charges, you would have no more responsibility in this matter.

Should such practitioners come to the attention of an ethics board, they usually need education or counseling and can return to an ethical practice without severe punishment or losing their license. In most instances, if it is a minor infraction, the therapist is ordered to attend additional hours of continuing education in ethics, pay a fine, and sometimes have a temporary suspension of his or her license.

Dealing with Predatory Behavior

If there are persistent rumors about a practitioner taking sexual advantage of clients, or if a client has come to you for help with making a complaint, you may want to get involved out of concern for the clients and the reputation of the profession. You need to let clients know that taking action against a predator isn't easy. As in other professions, such suits usually involve female clients and male practitioners. Female clients who have been harassed or mistreated sometimes wrongly feel that they colluded with the predator and are ashamed to take action. Also, women who are taken in by predators are frequently already emotionally fragile and may not make good witnesses. The accusers themselves—either the victims or those acting on their behalf—can become the target of either hostility or legal action from the accused or his supporters.

Taking someone to court or filing a complaint with the massage board is time-consuming and emotionally wrenching. The majority of massage boards do not take action on anonymous complaints, which is a double-edged sword. Like a court of law, the underlying principle there is that an accused person has the right to face their accuser; the downside is that many people won't come forward, so a predator may get away with illegal and devastating behavior if no one is willing to come forward. Those pursuing such a complaint are performing a service both for the profession and for future would-be victims of that practitioner.

Confusion and Imperfection

Because of the public's misconceptions, manual therapists have to make an extra effort to combat the public misconception that links our work with sexual services.

However, we don't need to go too far in the other direction and have unrealistic expectations of ourselves—for instance, to expect ourselves never to have even fleeting sexual thoughts about our clients. We need to be able to be honest with ourselves and each other about our mistakes and humanness.

The sexual issues related to our work can be potentially problematic for manual therapists, as individual practitioners and as a profession. Misunderstandings, inappropriate behavior, and accusations related to sex are the most damaging to both the practitioner and the profession. How do we lower the risk and keep our work environment safe for ourselves and therapeutic for our clients? We should seek outside professional help when we need more clarity about sexual issues that interfere with our work. We need to have more honest discussion among fellow students and colleagues. And we need to soften our attitudes so that we can allow for imperfection and confusion in ourselves and others, while stopping the behaviors that harm clients.

Questions for Reflection

1. If you are a manual therapist or studying to be one, do you have any fears about sexual issues related to this work? What could you do to lessen those fears?

2. Imagine how a female practitioner might feel while working with a new male client who appears to be having an erection. What would her concerns be? How might she act? Imagine how a man might feel who finds himself having an erection while he is getting a massage from a woman practitioner he does not know well. What would his concerns be? How might he act?

3. Have you ever known of a professional of any kind who was habitually sexually inappropriate or habitually seduced his or her clients? How would you feel about reporting such a person to his or her professional association? What would make you hesitate? What would make you want to go forward?

4. How would it feel to have people assume that because you are a man, a homosexual, or a person of color, you might be more sexually aggressive or less trustworthy than other people? What would you do to combat that image? What could you do to not take it personally?

5. Do you think you could be easily attracted to a client who acts seductively? Or could you imagine circumstances in your life (being lonely, feeling unsure of yourself because of a recent rejection, and so on) that would make you more vulnerable to such a client? What could you do to keep yourself from acting on such an attraction?

thePoint To learn more about the concepts discussed in this chapter, visit http://thePoint .lww.com/Allen-McIntosh4e

9

Financial Boundaries: Getting Comfortable with Money

Many practitioners in our profession are uneasy about the financial side of our work. Many of us come to this work without formal training in business or a business background. We spend much of our time in school learning our trade, not learning how to deal with money and fees. However, making sure the financial part of our relationship with clients is handled with clarity and grace is an important way that we set safe boundaries for our clients and ourselves.

We may think of the business side of the professional relationship as an unpleasant bit of reality that we tack on to the "true" relationship, the hands-on aspect of our work. But charging a fee (or whatever we ask in return for our work) is actually central to the therapeutic relationship. For the professional relationship to feel safe to clients, they need to know what we expect of them and they need to trust that we will be fair. Also, for the relationship to feel right to us, we need to feel that we are receiving adequate compensation.

This chapter discusses personal issues and attitudes practitioners can have about charging fees that may get in the way of creating effective financial transactions. It is primarily concerned with choices based on individual preference rather than on questions of business ethics.

CONSIDER THIS

Many massage therapists graduate from school with debt from student loans to repay. Many also enter with the "I just want to help people" attitude. That's a noble attitude, but it's hard to help others when you are worried about how to pay your rent or your car payment. Having clear financial policies, rather than alienating clients, will actually make your boundaries in this area clear to them, and help safeguard your own financial prosperity.

It is also primarily aimed at those who have or want to have a private practice. Of course, those who work for others have concerns about financial compensation as well. If you choose to work for someone else, your main task is to make sure the financial arrangements are fair to you before you start employment. For instance, you would want to know whether you are paid if a client cancels at the last minute, how much you are paid for downtime, how you will receive your tips, or what else you might be required to do, such as cleaning or laundry. A good book on business practices would be useful.

From Caring One to Cashier: Money Awkwardness

Some of us may feel awkward going from being the one who is compassionate when a client is on the table to being the one who asks for money at the end of the session.

> ➤ *You've just finished a session during which you felt touched by a client's revelation of the pain he feels in his life, and you're feeling compassionate toward him. As he gets ready to pay, he says, "Oh, do you mind if I postdate this check for next week?" or "Gee, I forgot my checkbook. Mind if I pay you next time?" How do you then say, "I prefer that you pay me at the end of each session," without feeling callous? It might seem easier to say, "Oh, sure . . . that's fine," even if it really isn't fine.*

Caring about clients and expecting something in return from them are two different aspects of our relationship with our clients, and we may feel uncomfortable making the transition between the two. Medical doctors and other practitioners who do volume business resolve the conflict by having another person, an office manager or a receptionist, handle the finances. If you work for someone else, your employer generally has office staff that takes care of the business end. But those who are in private practice are stuck with the dilemma of sliding back and forth between being the caring one and the cashier.

Perhaps we even feel a little guilty about setting fees. A bodyworker said recently, "I'm not in this for the money. This work is like a calling for me." For those with that attitude, there's often an accompanying sentiment that it's somehow crass to care about making money. While there's nothing wrong with wanting to make the world a better, there's also nothing wrong with being paid adequately for our work. Part of what being a professional means, after all, is that this is how we pay the rent. Charging appropriate fees tells clients that we respect ourselves and are serious about our work.

For practitioners who are uncomfortable because they feel as if they're charging people for nurturing them or caring about them, a colleague has this advice: "Tell them that clients are paying for their time. The caring is free."

CONSIDER THIS

We all have obligations we have to meet. Food, shelter, clothing, utilities, medical care, child care, student loan debt; the list goes on. Those who have children often have worries about how they are going to pay for their education or how they would cope in the event of some unforeseen financial catastrophe. In addition to the necessities, most people want to be able to take an occasional vacation, put money in savings for a rainy day, plan for their retirement, and be able to give something to their favorite charities. The desire to be in service, and help people through massage, doesn't need to exclude the realities of making a comfortable living. If you're independently wealthy, don't need to worry about making money, and truly want to give away your services, then carry on, but if you're like the majority who have real needs that they need to take care of, and the occasional wants, then you have to be realistic about your financial boundaries and how to handle those with clients.

On the other hand, if you have entered this profession because you think it's an easy way to make a living and don't realize the need for a caring attitude, you will find the work challenging in a different way. I've met many therapists over the years who work second jobs to make ends meet, or who end up leaving the profession altogether because they cannot sustain themselves with the amount of income they make.

Money As Part of the Healing Process

For those who are shy about charging, you have to keep in mind that your fees or compensation is actually an important part of the healing process for clients. Our fees clarify clients' obligations to us and ours to them. Giving a service without making it clear what we expect in return can make both parties uneasy.

It is an intrinsic aspect of clients' healing not only for them to give something in return but also to create a balance by giving something that is valuable to them. In *Persuasion and Healing*, the authors studied many kinds of health-care providers—witch doctors, traditional Western medical doctors, and alternative health practitioners. They concluded that in an effective therapeutic experience, patients or clients must give something valuable in exchange; they must make a sacrifice (Frank JD, Frank JB. *Persuasion and Healing*. Baltimore, MD: Johns Hopkins University Press; 1993). In cultures other than our own, the offering might be a nice fat chicken. In ours, it might be someone volunteering their time so that a new student

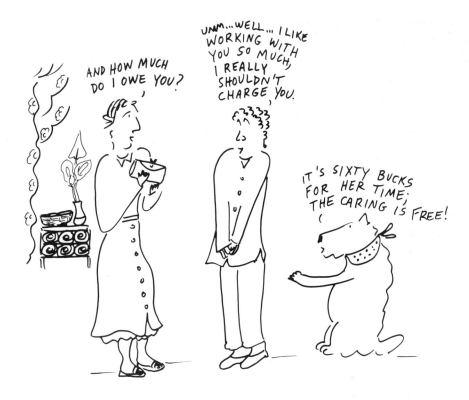

can practice on them or a colleague trading a session. However, usually what is given is money.

The idea of the healing value of a sacrifice doesn't justify greed or overcharging, but the concept can help us feel more comfortable with collecting appropriate fees. The element of sacrifice may give clients a deeper sense of the treatment's value and help them benefit from it. Sometimes clients who are given a special deal don't seem to get as much out of the work as those who pay full price.

Although trades can occasionally work out well, money is usually the best way to be compensated. The great thing about money is that it's specific. Sixty dollars isn't the same as $59.75. Money's clean; it's precise; it's simple.

Money's clean; it is precise; it is simple.

The clarity of fees is part of a safe professional environment. It is useful to both practitioner and client. Asking for and receiving money (or whatever the terms of exchange) speaks deeply to both client and practitioner about the value of the work. For practitioners, money is a tangible sign of the client's appreciation. For clients, it is a tangible sign of how much they will invest in their own well-being.

REAL EXPERIENCE

Early in my career, I learned a few lessons about doing trades and bartering for massage. I made one barter arrangement with a carpet and window cleaner that has worked out well for over a decade now, but in other situations, I haven't been as fortunate. I made one deal with a painter that turned out badly; I was so dissatisfied with the sloppy job they did in repainting my office, I ultimately ended up paying someone else to do it. I made another exchange with someone who agreed to do weekly housecleaning, and that just turned out horribly—she was constantly calling with excuses why she couldn't come in to do it when she was scheduled. After a few weeks of her constant rescheduling, I just gave up on that. With the exception of my reliable carpet cleaner, which is a trade that just happens a couple of times a year, I have found that things work out better when I just pay the money for the services I need, and collect the money from the people I give services to.

—L.K., LMT

Money: An Emotional Issue

As we all know, money can be an emotionally-loaded issue. Most people have strong beliefs, opinions, and habits around money. Very few people are indifferent to the subject. The fact that both practitioner and client may have strong feelings and attitudes about money makes it both more important and more challenging to keep consistent boundaries in this area.

Regardless of their actual material wealth, some clients may be concerned about whether they are getting their money's worth. They may be sensitive to being slighted on time or effort. They may think our fees are too high. Perhaps not being aware of the expenses of running a small business or the physical and emotional exertion that our work involves, they may think a professional who makes $80 an hour is lavishly paid. Or they may take our fee setting personally, thinking that we don't like them if we raise our fees and we do like them if we give them a discount. (We have to be careful that the latter isn't true and that discounts are based on objective criteria.)

Some of us may have old, unexamined ideas that get in the way of making good decisions about policies concerning money and fees. We might have deep feelings about whether money is "good" or "bad," whether we are competent with it, or even whether we deserve to be financially successful. Sometimes, this is related to the attitudes and financial circumstances we were raised in. Someone who grew up in a home that struggled in their financial circumstances is apt to have a much different attitude about money than someone who grew up in a well-to-do family.

We might have unrealistic ideas about how hard or how easy it is to make a living; unfortunately, many massage school students are told that "you'll get out of school and immediately be making $75 an hour!" or similar rubbish. Truthfully, we work in a profession that usually doesn't make us rich. In a culture that measures personal worth by one's bank account, we have to learn to value our work nonetheless.

Talking to Clients About Money

Because money is an emotional subject for many people, we can quickly offend or even lose a client if we are clumsy in setting limits or unclear about our expectations around fee paying.

Here is a summary of the basic guidelines for setting limits for any practitioner who has to explain financial expectations to clients. These were first discussed in Chapter 6:

- Be clear about expectations in advance.
- Be careful about your tone.
- Speak in terms of your general policy.
- Practice what you will say in various situations.

The importance of these guidelines is worth repeating. First, the clearer you are about what you expect from the beginning, the easier your job will be. Second, when you talk with clients about money policies, your attitude and tone make a world of difference. You want to sound straightforward, businesslike, and confident—neither apologetic nor punitive. Third, when you have to set a limit, if you speak in terms of general policies rather than about a client's specific behavior or circumstances, the client will be less defensive. Avoid making it sound like a personal issue. Instead of saying, "You should have let me know you couldn't come. You have to pay me for the appointment you missed," you can say, perhaps with a sympathetic tone, "As it states on the office policies that we gave you during your first visit, I charge full fee when someone misses an appointment. I can always fill your appointment with another client if I have notice you need to cancel.

The ability to set limits well doesn't come naturally. Just as you use friends and colleagues to practice massage strokes, you can also use them to try out what you will say in different situations. Even though it's a make-believe situation, friends and family can give you valuable feedback about how your words sound and your attitude comes across.

Basic Fee Policies

There are a number of common situations or practices that most practitioners in private practice have to deal with around fee setting. As with other aspects of your relationship with clients, it's a good idea to establish fair boundaries and stick with them unless you have a carefully thought-out reason to make an exception. You also need to be familiar with the appropriate laws in your city or state to be sure you are in compliance with regulations governing various aspects of running a business, such as refund policies, raising fees, marketing, expiration dates on gift certificates (yes, this is regulated), and so forth. In the event you are working in a state that allows insurance billing for massage, or are accepting personal injury or Workman's Comp cases, bear in mind that you cannot bill for missed appointments on any type of insurance, but you may try to collect it from the client. Of course, if you work in a spa or as the employee of a doctor or chiropractor, you have to abide by their basic fee policies. As discussed earlier, it's a good idea to find out whether the employer's policies are agreeable to you before you take a job. Even one missed appointment may make a difference to a therapist who is on a tight budget, and if several people in a week miss an appointment and are not charged, your salary can dwindle pretty quickly.

Setting Fees

If you're starting a practice, you can determine the appropriate fee to charge by researching what other practitioners in your community are charging, especially those who offer your kind of bodywork or massage and have your level of experience.

Your rates affect what both clients and colleagues will think about you. If you charge noticeably more than the norm, some clients may be put off, while others may think you must be offering something special for the extra charge. If you charge substantially less than the going rate, some clients may be attracted to the bargain but may not value the work as much.

You must also consider how colleagues in the massage therapy profession will view you. If you are charging way less than the other therapists in your area, they may perceive that you are just trying to steal business by undercutting them. Competition is a healthy thing, but alienating every other massage therapist in the area is not. You may need someone to refer clients to in the future, or be in need of a massage yourself. It's best to practice friendly competition without using cutthroat business practices.

Sometimes even a $10 difference in fees can set a practitioner apart. Colleagues may feel you are arrogant if you charge more than they do without having more training or experience. On the other hand, it's more acceptable to offer discounted rates in order to boost business if you are a recent graduate, a practitioner new to an area, or even an experienced practitioner whose practice is in a slump. And surroundings do make a difference. A practitioner who works at home, or doing outcalls, does not have the same overhead as the therapist who rents a nice office in a professional building, but that doesn't mean their time and skills are less valuable. There is a lot to consider.

The amount you charge also affects how you feel about your work. Make sure that your fees are fair to you and that they take into account all of your expenses—for instance, your office rent; travel expense if you're doing outcalls; the time and cost of either laundering your own sheets or having them cleaned; and the costs of advertising, taxes, massage oil, phone service, or a website and all the other expenses that come with operating a business. Charge enough so that you won't begin to resent your clients. Also, make sure you don't feel as if you are overcharging. If you're not comfortable with your fees, clients will sense it and feel uncomfortable also.

Raising Fees

How often and by how much practitioners raise their fees can vary. Many raise their fees by $5 or $10 about once a year. Some raise rates when their overhead, such as office rent, becomes higher. To be fair, you need to give adequate notice—a month or two, at least—to let clients get used to the idea of the higher rate and be able to budget accordingly. You can post a notice by your door so that clients will be sure to see it, mail or e-mail a notice to your regular clients, post it on your website, send it out in your newsletter if you have one. You can also tell them (before they are on the table): "I want to let you know that starting in November, my fee will be $65 instead of $60."

There's a good deal of variation in how you can carry out fee hikes. Some practitioners begin charging the higher fee immediately for new clients but wait a month or two before applying the rate for existing clients. Some never raise rates for existing clients; their clients never pay more than what they paid for in their first appointment.

There's no set way to raise fees. Whatever you decide, your policy needs to be one that you can live with, that you feel is fair to you and to your clients, and that you implement consistently. There's no need to feel apologetic about raising your fees. As a colleague said, "We don't need to send clients a sympathy card when we raise our fees."

Special Deals

What about giving discounts or using sliding scales? Most of the practitioners I have talked with find it works best to stick with one fee, with rare exceptions.

As discussed in earlier chapters, making special arrangements for a client in any area of your work generally brings up a red flag. Because money issues are often so emotionally loaded for both client and practitioner, going outside your usual boundaries in fee setting is often a big mistake. It can also be a sign of deeper problems with your professional relationship with a client; you may be allowing the client to manipulate you.

Giving discounts and charging on a sliding scale that depends on the client's income are the most common examples of special deals. A colleague reports:

➤ *A prospective client called and said she was under a lot of stress, and she knew it would help her to receive regular massages. She had heard good things about my work but said that massage was "outside her budget" and asked if I would give her a significant discount. Since she was working full time, I told her that I only offered discounts to senior citizens. When she began pleading with me about how much she needed the work, I almost gave in to her, but then realized that I was inappropriately beginning to take on responsibility for her stress level. I told her that I couldn't make an exception for her, suggested that she might go to the clinic of the local massage school, and I gave her the names of a newly graduated practitioner who might be willing to give her a discount. Although she was not happy about being refused, I felt that she had not given me a good reason to change my policies—and she had given me good reason to be wary of being manipulated.*

You're under no obligation to discount your fees. In many ways, charging everyone the same fee creates the safest, clearest boundaries for both you and your clients. If you do want to consider discounting your fees or making special arrangements from time to time, consider the following points:

Know Your Motivation

You want to take care that, for one, you're not trying to rescue the client. A "rescue" attitude means you treat the client as if they were in some way inadequate and, therefore, not able to be held to normal business arrangements. Sometimes you may make a special deal because you don't want to say no to a client, you want to be "nice," or you think you need the money, even if it's a lower fee. All of these motivations are different from making an adult-to-adult business arrangement with someone who has a legitimate reason to need a discount, such as an elderly person on a small fixed income. Equally important, when you depart from your normal framework, you encourage clients to do so as well. A colleague reports:

➤ *Even though I don't usually do this, I made a special payment arrangement for a client who said he was down on his luck. He was to receive a 10-session series at the rate of two per month but was to pay me for only one each month. After we finished the 10th session, he would continue to pay me a monthly fee until all sessions were paid off. Unfortunately, once we started working, I found that he was an inconsiderate client. For instance, he was often late to sessions, even after I urged him to be on time. Once he missed a session without giving adequate cancellation notice. When we were finished with our work, I had a hard time collecting what he owed me. Lesson learned. I had started out badly with this client by making a special fee arrangement without good cause. By not respecting my own professional boundaries, I had encouraged him to not respect them either.*

You can avoid confusion if you have clear guidelines concerning the circumstances under which you will make a special arrangement.

Offer Discounts to Groups of People, Not Individuals

Those who do offer discounts often restrict them to certain groups of people, rather than deciding merit on an individual basis. Some school clinics and private practitioners, for example, offer discounts or pro bono work to veterans, elderly people on a small fixed income, people with life-threatening illnesses, or spiritual or religious teachers. A special fee can work well if it's motivated by your heart or your convictions and not by guilt.

A special fee can work well if it's motivated by your heart or your convictions and not by guilt.

When you make such an exception, you need to keep checking in with yourself to make sure your heart is still in it and your bank balance isn't suffering.

Be Wary of Sliding Scales

Using a sliding scale to determine fees means that you offer a range of fees based on the client's income. For instance, someone who has a low salary would pay your lowest rate of $40 per hour and a wealthier person would pay your standard rate of $90 an hour, with gradations in between. Sliding scales are basically discounts, so you need to employ the same caution about using them. Using a sliding scale to determine fees based on a client's statement about his ability to pay automatically creates a dual relationship. In a sense, you become the client's banker, involving yourself in his finances in ways that aren't supposed to be part of your role. For instance, you may find yourself concerned about whether the client is spending his money wisely in other areas of his life or whether you should renegotiate his fee if his income rises. The complications created by going outside the boundaries of the therapeutic relationship in this way can interfere with the relationship and with your ability to put your best effort into your work. Imagine these scenarios:

➤ *A client has convinced you that, as a student, she can't afford your full fee. You have agreed to accept $50 per session instead of your usual $80 fee. After you've seen her for a couple of months, she tells you she can't make her appointments* *for the next few weeks because she's going to a concert and "had to pay $200 for the ticket!". How do you feel?*

➤ *A client who is paying you less than full fee complains after several sessions that she's not getting enough from the work, that she doesn't feel as good as she wants to. Would you be able to handle this complaint with the same objectivity as you would if she were a full-fee client, or might you secretly feel that she's being ungrateful?*

➤ *A client who has been receiving a discounted fee arrives for her session in a new car—a much more expensive model than the one you drive yourself. When you mention it, she says "yes, I've always wanted one so I saved up for the down payment." Do you feel that you contributed to her ability to save for a fancy car by discounting your fee?*

Ask Yourself Some Pointed Questions

Even if you offer to do pro bono or discounted work for what seems like purely altruistic reasons, you want to look at the difficulties that may be hidden in such relationships. Here are some good questions to ask yourself any time you consider reducing fees:

- Do I have a standard policy for fee reduction, and am I veering from that policy?
- Am I reluctant to say no to this client?
- How do I decide how much of a discount to give?
- What are the possibilities that the special financial arrangement will affect the therapeutic relationship?
- Am I expecting special gratitude and appreciation in return for this special fee?

Monitor the Number of Discounted-Fee Arrangements You Have at One Time

Determine how many discounted or pro bono (no fee) clients you can realistically afford to see in your practice at one time. You don't want to work all week and end up with little cash to show for it.

It's difficult to make blanket statements about when it's appropriate to give a discount. Some practitioners can handle giving discounts and making special arrangements more easily than others. In deciding what policies you are comfortable with, you have to be honest with yourself about your own limit-setting abilities and your own feelings and biases about money. The bottom line is to consider honestly whether the arrangement could be detrimental to you, your client, or the professional relationship.

Common Financial Dilemmas

A number of common situations that arise in the work life of a somatic practitioner in private practice can create difficulties. Although solutions to the problems may vary from practitioner to practitioner, it's best for each practitioner to establish his or her own policy for each of these situations and then stay with that policy.

Missed Appointments

You've booked a new client at 3 p.m. You're not at the movies, you're not taking a nap, you're not attending a class. And most important, you're not able to schedule another client for that time slot. You're all prepared: you've warmed up the room, put clean sheets on the table. Maybe you were counting on the money and you've already mentally spent the fee. And then . . . no client. No phone messages to explain . . . nothing. The missed appointment is that dreadful thud in the professional life of a manual therapist.

The missed appointment is that dreadful thud in the professional life of a manual therapist.

Along with the dreadful thud goes the pesky question of whether to ask the client to pay for the missed session. If the client had a genuine emergency, you wouldn't charge. But what constitutes an authentic emergency? Certainly, someone's child breaking an arm is a genuine crisis, and it's understandable that they'd rush off to the emergency room instead of thinking about your appointment. Sometimes no-show clients truly can't anticipate problems, but often they can. Illness rarely comes on so suddenly that they wouldn't have the time to call and tell you they aren't coming. Business people usually know that meetings can run long. It's hard to know where to draw the line.

In most circumstances, standard practice is to charge a full or partial fee for someone who breaks an appointment without adequate notice or just doesn't show up. (Manual therapists sometimes make exceptions and don't charge the first time a client misses an appointment.) Some practitioners—especially new ones—find it hard to ask a client to pay for a missed appointment. They feel awkward asking payment for "doing nothing." The point is that you could have booked another client in that slot, and even if no other clients wanted that time period, you lost the time it took to prepare and the 20 minutes or so it took to determine that the client wasn't coming. A missed appointment is time and money lost. Also, if you allow clients to be disrespectful of your time once, chances are they will do it again.

Sometimes practitioners are concerned about making the client angry, so they rationalize that they wouldn't have filled the vacancy anyway. But you have to consider whether you want to work with a client who doesn't respect your time. Also, if you are angry with a client for missing appointments without notice, can you be compassionate when you work with that client? If you're resentful of their treatment of you, that's likely to come through in your attitude with them.

Sticking to your guns about charging for missed appointments shows that you value your time as a professional. Unfortunately, if the no-show client doesn't call either to explain or to make another appointment and won't return your calls, obviously you can't do anything about it. Such a client probably wouldn't respond to a written bill, either.

To be fair about the adequate-notice policy, you should show clients the same courtesy. Let them know that if you have to cancel an appointment without 24-hour notice, you will give them a free or discounted session. Even with a firm policy that has been communicated to clients, most practitioners have an occasional no-show. Here are some suggestions to make missed appointments less frequent:

Set Your Policy When the First Appointment Is Made

When a client schedules a first appointment, always make sure you let her or him know you will charge for appointments cancelled without 24-hour cancellation notice (or whatever you think is adequate).

Put It in Writing

- During the first appointment, ask clients to sign an agreement accepting the 24-hour cancellation policy (and whatever other policies you have, such as being paid at the time of the session). Even if you are certain you have told clients, they may not remember that you did.

- Be sure to include in this agreement the amount of time you will wait—for instance, 15 or 20 minutes or whatever you feel comfortable with—before you decide that the appointment has been missed. Let clients know that it's possible that you might leave the office at that point, so that even if they do finally show up, they may not be able to have even a partial session.

- Have your cancellation policy on your website, your brochures, your intake form, a sign in your lobby...make it so visible that people can't possibly miss it.

Confirm Your Appointments

Ask permission to call or text the client with a reminder a day or two in advance of the appointment. Giving clients an appointment card is helpful, but if they stick that in their purse or wallet, they may forget it's there. It's a good idea for clients to get used to having standing appointments, whether that's once a week or once a month. It will help them to remember that every Monday at 4 p.m., they'll be seeing you.

Many therapists are using online scheduling now, which can be set to automatically send clients reminders of their appointments.

Explore Credit Card Payments

If you are able to take credit card payments, you can ensure payment in the way that other businesses, such as hotels, do. When a client makes an appointment, take her or his credit card number and let the client know you will charge for a missed session unless the appointment is cancelled by a certain time. Using the credit card method is particularly useful for those who work a great deal with one-time clients, such as vacationers in resort towns. Many of the previously mentioned online schedulers require the credit card before confirmation of the appointment.

Gift Certificates

Some practitioners offer gift certificates as a way to promote business or bring in extra income, especially around the holidays. While they can bring in extra income, gift certificates can also bring some problems.

Many experienced practitioners say that gift certificates are often not worth the trouble. For instance, the giver of the gift may be much more enthusiastic about the benefits of massage than the recipient; the recipient may be reluctant, for whatever reason, to have a massage. As a result, recipients sometimes drag their feet about collecting their massage. Sometimes as much as a year can pass before they make an appointment. Because of this, some practitioners put an expiration date on gift certificates. However, most practitioners say they wouldn't turn down such a client regardless of when she or he calls.

Federal law enacted in 2009 requires that gift certificates must be honored for 5 years. Some states are more restrictive than the federal law, and require that they not have an expiration date at all, in which case you are obligated to abide by the more restrictive law. You may find the information about your state at www.ncsl.org/research/financial-services-and-commerce/gift-cards-and-certificates-statutes-and-legis.aspx.

Although there are these downsides to gift certificates, they work well for some practitioners. And for some, the process of advertising and selling gift certificates is a good exercise in learning how to promote their businesses.

Extreme Deals

The Internet abounds with companies such as Groupon, Living Social, and other sites that businesses can use to promote themselves. You agree to discount your services very steeply on these sites—maybe even as much as 75% off. In exchange, the site keeps a portion of the sales, which buyers must pay for on the site, and they advertise your deal to their subscribers in your area. You may set a limit on how many deals you can offer and when they expire—because it's a discount—not a gift certificate.

Some therapists have reported being satisfied with the results they realized from participating, while others felt that the new people who came in were just chronic shoppers for cheap deals who would come once to get that $20 massage and never come again.

You need to be extremely careful about your participation in such deals, because you may find yourself giving months' worth of discounted massage and cutting substantially into your income. You also need to ask potential employers if they participate in such steep discounting, and if you will be paid your normal rate of pay for such deals, or if they plan to pass that steep discounting on to you in the form of a pay cut.

Refunds

It's often wise to offer a dissatisfied client a full or partial refund even if there has been no negligence or harm on your part. If a client is upset enough to ask for his money back, you're generally better off honoring that request. Aside from wanting to respect the client's wishes, you don't want the bad publicity of an angry ex-client complaining about you to others, especially now that so many people leave reviews on the Internet.

If a client has an unpleasant experience during a session, whether or not you were totally responsible, then you want to make it up to the client. Regardless of whether you had control over the situation that caused a client's discomfort, you bear some of the responsibility. Also, if you want to stay on good terms with the client, refunding all or part of a fee and offering a discount on a future session are good options. Here are two examples:

➤ *A massage therapist charged a client for only half a session when the last 20 minutes of the hour were disrupted by the loud barking of the neighbor's dog.*

➤ *A practitioner gave a total refund to a client who had had an allergic reaction to his scented massage oil. Although the client had not told the practitioner that she was sensitive to perfumes, the practitioner was still sorry that the client had had a bad experience and didn't want the client to have a negative feeling about his work.*

Certainly, if it *is* your fault that the client feels dissatisfied, you need to offer a full or partial refund:

➤ *A woman had received four sessions from a bodyworker. The bodyworker ended the fifth one 20 minutes earlier than the others, and the client felt the quality of the work was below what she'd come to expect. After leaving the bodyworker's office, she realized she felt shortchanged and called him, explaining what she had noticed. He told her that she was right—that he had been on the verge of catching the flu when he worked with her. He didn't explain that at the time— most clients would have been understanding, if the therapist said "I'm sorry, but I'm not feeling well. If we can cut this short now, I'll make it up to you during the next session." He did not apologize or offer a refund or a discount, or offer to make up the time on another session. Not surprisingly, the client never went back to him and never referred anyone else to him.*

This example doesn't mean that whenever you feel you've performed less than your best, you should rush to offer a free session. Those who are very self-critical would be constantly offering free sessions. However, it was the practitioner's responsibility to monitor his own energy level and health and cancel the appointment to avoid giving an inadequate session (and in this case, to avoid the possibility of giving the client the flu).

To steer clear of an irate client making a complaint to your professional association or filing a lawsuit, you may need to make it clear in writing that in giving the refund you are not admitting that you have been in the wrong. Also, along with acknowledging receipt of the refund, you may want the client to agree in writing to take no further action and make no further complaints against you. If you have doubts about how best to make a refund without giving the client fuel for further action, you would be wise to get professional legal counsel. Some therapists go so far as to have a clause on their intake form about arbitration, in the event the client is dissatisfied to the point of wanting money refunded.

Gratuities and Gifts

Whether to accept gratuities (tips) and whether to accept gifts are two other common money issues and affect both those in private practice and those who are employed.

Gratuities

Whether or not to accept gratuities can be a controversial subject for somatic practitioners. Some practitioners question whether it's professional for massage therapists to accept tips because other professionals do not. Most think that practitioners who work for themselves should charge adequate fees and not accept tips. However, for those who work for lower wages in a spa or salon, tips can be a necessary financial supplement.

There are ways to make the tipping issue less confusing and awkward for clients. Customers who receive a massage in a spa or salon often aren't sure whether

After the first professional massage I ever received as a client, I was unsure of the protocol, so I asked if she accepted tips. She said "The best tip you can give me is to refer someone else to me." She's still my therapist 10 years later, and I have referred many people to her. When I made a mid-life career change and became a massage therapist myself just a couple of years ago, I decided to have the same policy. A tip is nice, but referrals are better—more business—and I think clients may look at me more as a member of their health-care team because I don't accept tips.

—M.H., MT

to tip. The owners may make their tipping policy clear by posting a sign on the premises or adding a statement on their list of services: "Gratuities are appreciated," and having a gratuity line on their credit card slips.

When the practice of tipping is encouraged in a spa or salon or other setting with more than one therapist, it's best if there's an envelope for each employee at the check-in desk (and that the clients know that) so that a practitioner won't necessarily know how much a particular client has given and can concentrate on doing a good job for *all* clients. Clients may prefer that the therapist *does* know who left it for them, because they want the therapist to know that they appreciated them.

Gifts

Gifts from clients are a more personal sign of appreciation than tips. Whether to accept gifts needs to be evaluated on a case-by-case basis, taking into consideration the size and value of the gift and what the client's intention seems to be.

It's *not okay* to pressure clients for tips, or to give them less service and attention because they're not good tippers. I've had many therapists over the years ask me how they can let clients know they "expect" a tip, and in some cases, they've been blatant: "How can I let my clients know I expect a $20 tip?" My suggestion is that you set your fees at the amount of money you really want—and do not "expect" a tip—ever.

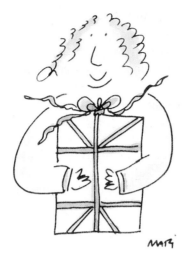

Inexpensive gifts given on holidays or special occasions as signs of clients' affection or appreciation are generally fine to accept. You might think twice, however, about accepting frequent gifts, larger gifts, or gifts that you know are an extravagance for the client. Also, if you are uncertain about the intention behind the gift—for instance, if you know a client is interested in dating you and may want to win you over—it would be best to refuse the gift. Clients who give lavish gifts may, at some level, hope for some special treatment in return. Suppose a client gave you an expensive gift and then wanted the work to continue past the end of the hour.

If you want to refuse a gift for whatever reason, you may do so with a smile and a firm, "Thank you for thinking of me, but I really can't accept this." Whether to give discounts or refunds, offer gift certificates, or take tips are questions that practitioners have to decide for themselves. Whatever your decision, it always needs to be with an eye toward creating clear and comfortable boundaries for yourself and your clients. The question to ask yourself always has to be the same: "Could this action harm the therapeutic relationship?"

Rewards for Referrals

Is it a good business practice to reward clients or other professionals for referring clients to you in hopes of stimulating more referrals?

Here are two examples:

➤ *Massage therapist Margaret offers a free massage to any client who refers five new clients who make and keep an appointment with her.*

➤ *Bodyworker Bruce has an arrangement with a chiropractor (for whom Bruce does not work) to give the chiropractor $10 for each new client the chiropractor refers.*

In many jurisdictions, these practices are known as "kickbacks" and are illegal as they are considered unethical and unprofessional. Prospective clients need to be able to assume that the person recommending you is doing so because he or she appreciates your competence and skill, not because he or she is getting a fee or a reward of any kind in return. Even though the referrer may appreciate your abilities, the reward can influence his or her judgment.

As a professional, you should expect that clients and other professionals will find your work valuable and want to tell others about it. Although you want to be courteous and thank them for any referrals, a professional should not be in the position of seeming overly grateful for a referral, and when you are not rewarding the referrer, that is an assurance that they feel grateful for having a skilled and trustworthy practitioner to whom to refer friends and colleagues. On top of a verbal thank you, people really appreciate getting a handwritten thank you card. That is sufficient—and not unethical.

Becoming More Comfortable with Money

Sometimes we graduate from our manual therapy training expecting that we should be able to easily make a good living with our work. However, it may take a while for this expectation to become a reality, and we can feel isolated in grappling with the situation. It's rare for people to share the details of their financial struggles with others, so we may not realize that other practitioners are often having the same problems.

It's not unusual for practitioners to occasionally make mistakes in dealing with clients about money, especially when just starting out in business. At some point in their careers, most practitioners have backed down from charging a client for an appointment cancelled at the last minute, for example, or have given a special discount that backfired, or have undercharged or overcharged a client.

There are ways that we can become more secure with financial dealing. We can first examine our own attitudes about money. Having **mentors** who are comfortable in their relationship to money can be a major help with business issues. Because just about everyone has some issues about money and business, peer group discussions can also be helpful. In a group, others will have clarity about issues that we struggle with. Consultations with a professional counselor can also aid us in getting to the deeper issues that we have about money. (Peer groups and consultations are discussed more fully in Chapter 12.)

Mentor:
A trusted colleague who provides guidance and education. Mentors are usually helpful in advising on both the details of establishing oneself as a professional and the broader general aspects of taking on a professional role or of taking on the role of a particular kind of bodywork or massage practitioner.

Some manual therapists are starting to use coaches—individuals specifically trained to help practitioners create business goals that suit their values. A coach can help us figure out the steps to reach those goals and then, like a personal exercise trainer, hold us accountable for making progress. However, be choosy about choosing a coach! Someone who has actually been the proprietor of their own business is apt to know more about the realities of business than someone who just took training in being a coach.

Some workshops specialize in improving attitudes about money. To find a good workshop or coach, seek out recommendations from satisfied customers. For practical advice and legal information, it's useful to attend a workshop, such as one at a local community college, about how to run a small business. Many Chambers of Commerce, as well as the Small Business Administration, and local merchant's associations often sponsor such classes.

The ability to set good money boundaries is a crucial part of our work. Clients need the comfort and safety of a clear financial relationship, and so do we. Keeping clean and clear about money is, like most boundary issues, a skill and an art that we will practice and improve throughout our careers.

Questions for Reflection

1. Fill in the blank with the first words or phrases that come to mind: In my life, money is _____. (You may have several answers.)

2. Think about how or where you may have gotten the feelings or thoughts about money that you wrote in question #1. Did they come from your family? From the culture? Do those answers reflect the attitude you want to have about money? If not, what attitude would you like to have? Fill in the blank to reflect that attitude: I want money to be _____.

3. Do you think it's true that clients will value a service according to what they pay for it? For instance, will they value a service they pay for more than a free one? Will they value a more expensive service more than a less expensive one? For instance, if a massage costs $10 rather than $60, will that make a difference in how the client perceives the service? Why or why not?

4. Draw up a list of money policies that you would be comfortable with as a practitioner. If you are already in practice, are there any changes you would make to your current policies?

thePoint To learn more about the concepts discussed in this chapter, visit http://thePoint .lww.com/Allen-McIntosh4e

CHAPTER 10

Dual Relationships and Boundaries: Wearing Many Hats

Dual relationships—having more than one kind of relationship with a client, such as being friends with a client or trading sessions with a colleague—are practically a tradition in our profession. We almost feel as if we have a right to them. Some of us become indignant at the thought of limiting or eliminating dual relationships: "What! I can't have coffee with a client?" "My buddy Bill has been coming to me for years, and it's just fine." "Where would I get clients if not from people I know?" However, many experienced therapists have discovered that such relationships can be more troublesome than they at first appear.

> **Dual relationships:**
> Having a relationship with a client other than the contractual therapeutic one, such as having a client who is also a friend, family member, or business associate.

Dual Relationships: Complicated Dynamics

Dual relationships can seem so easy—it can feel natural to become friends with a likable client. It can seem logical to work with friends and family—who better to share our gifts with than people we already love? However, the confusion of changing roles and the power of transference and countertransference can add complications.

When we try to become friends with Client Carrie, who knows you only as a selfless, always-caring massage therapist focused solely on Carrie's needs, it may be hard for her to get used to you as a regular person who is sometimes grumpy, insensitive, or needy herself. Or when Big Sister Sally, who knew you when you were throwing baby food on the floor, becomes Client Sally, she may have trouble taking you seriously and viewing you as a competent professional. With dual relationships, each person must shift back and forth between an existing role and a new one, and the transition is not always smooth. More often than not, it is messy and can lead to misunderstandings and stress in our practices.

Here's an example:

➤ *A massage therapist decided to barter with an old friend—she would give him massages, and he would wallpaper her living room. He wasn't a professional, but he said he could do a good job, and he was willing to do the exchange.*

As the work progressed, she became unhappy with both her own behavior and the client's. They both began treating sessions like social visits. She found herself talking about their mutual friends or her own concerns during sessions. His behavior was equally casual—he usually showed up late for his massage appointments and then made business calls on his cell phone before getting ready for the session. Because he was a friend, she had a hard time asserting herself about his loose time boundaries.

To make matters worse, she was unhappy with the quality of his work on her home. When he'd finished the living room, she told him that she felt his work was inadequate. He was surprised and offended when she pointed out flaws in the work. She ended up feeling dissatisfied, he felt offended when she said she should have hired a professional to begin with, and their friendship suffered.

We can't know all the reasons for this unhappy outcome, but it was no doubt complicated by the effects of transference. The client involved in the trade said later that he had become accustomed to seeing his friend as the nurturer. He had come to expect her to take care of him, forgetting that he had an adult responsibility for his side of the bargain. He then felt hurt when she criticized his work. When we are switching roles, the effects of transference and countertransference can create confusing situations.

In this story, we also see examples of two problems that are discussed later—how easy it is for both parties to be casual about framework when we are working with friends and the difficulty of **bartering** services or doing **trades**, especially with someone who is not trading his or her own professional services.

Many experienced practitioners stay clear of dual relationships because of the built-in problems. Whether we're trying to turn a client into a friend, doing a trade, or any of the other possibilities, both sides can end up feeling shortchanged.

Bartering:
Exchanging a manual therapy session for goods or services other than another manual therapy session.

Trade:
Exchanging a manual therapy session for a manual therapy session with a colleague.

Common Problems with Dual Relationships

Here are the most prevalent kinds of dual relationships and how they can be problematic.

Becoming Friends with Clients

It's not unusual for clients to want to become friends with us. Clients feel the heart connection in our work and want that connection to extend outside the sessions. We may feel the client's affection toward us and mistakenly think that affection should be carried into our daily lives rather than remain as part of the professional relationship, where it belongs. Or perhaps we find ourselves really liking a client and wanting to build that into a friendship. Despite those feelings, it's often a mistake to try to change the therapeutic relationship into a social one.

The effects of transference can make it hard to ever have an equal relationship. Because clients often give more weight to what we say and do, it may be unrealistic to expect them to adjust to the normal give and take of a friendship. On some level, clients usually have difficulty seeing us as real people with flaws and our own concerns. Even outside the office, they may expect us to be always focused on their needs, as we are during a session. There is also a chance that they would always see us as better or wiser than they are—and that we really are—and that we would exploit that in some way, even unconsciously.

Socializing with clients should occur rarely, if at all. Take an honest look at your friendships; if most of your friends are clients, then ask yourself how that came to be, and whether or not it's healthy for both you and the clients. The waters of the therapeutic relationship can get very muddied if we're not careful.

There is also the possibility that we would disappoint the client by showing our humanness. A colleague reports:

➤ *A client I had seen for several months asked me to have lunch with her, and we began to socialize. Prior to that, she had been an enthusiastic client—she saw massage as part of a new, healthier way of life, and she saw me as part of this new and exciting direction. Unfortunately, as she got to know me, she found out that I wasn't as perfect in my lifestyle as she had imagined—for instance, I declined several invitations to attend her church, and mentioned that I sometimes go to a hookah bar in town. She became disillusioned and discouraged and stopped making massage appointments.*

Befriending some of our clients can also interfere with our relationships with other clients. They may hear about these friendships and become jealous or uncomfortable about the limits of our boundaries.

Here are some guidelines for dealing with the temptation of becoming friends with clients:

Ask Yourself if the Change in Roles Would Benefit the Client

Be sure you're not using the client. When you're tempted to become friends with a client, ask yourself if changing the boundaries of the therapeutic relationship truly helps the client or primarily fulfills your own needs.

I moved halfway across the country with my husband when he got a job transfer. Our new home was a much smaller town than the city we had moved from, and there was no massage therapist in town. I got my new license, rented a small office space, and started to slowly build a clientele. People were friendly and when they found out I was new in town, they invited me to their churches, community potluck suppers, their parties, and social occasions. I soon found myself in the position of having several new friends who were all clients. In retrospect, I'm sure it was because I was in a strange place and lonely without my old circle of friends, but it was not without its problems. I found out that everybody knows everybody else's business. My office is on Main Street, and I couldn't go in the grocery store without someone saying "I saw Mary Jo coming out of your office today. Is she feeling better after having that nasty fall last week?" or other nosy questions and comments. I wasn't used to that, and when I would say "I can't talk about my clients," people would look at me like I'd sprouted horns. It was a big adjustment. The town was so small that there was really no way to avoid dual relationships, so I had to educate people about keeping my work life and my social life separate.

—J.G., CMT

Here is a colleague's experience:

➤ *I never socialize with my clients or even ex-clients, so I was surprised to find myself thinking about asking my client Mary to attend a concert with me. I realized that I was drawn to this unusual boundary bending because I was lonely. A good friend had recently moved away, and I had a gap in my social life. I felt tempted to fill it with a client I really liked. Once I realized what the problem was, I began thinking of other ways to find new friends.*

Evaluate Whether This Client Could Ever See You As an Equal

Honestly ask yourself whether the client could ever be a friend with you or whether that client has you on a pedestal. A colleague reports:

➤ *I was thinking of accepting the invitation of a client to attend a movie together. I liked this client and sensed that she wanted to be friends, but I was concerned that if she saw me in my day-to-day life, I might do something that would interfere with the professional relationship, such as saying something that would hurt her feelings. When I expressed my doubts to her, she said, "Oh, I know it'll be okay to be friends. I know you would never do anything that would be harmful to me." Her saying that helped me see how idealized I was in her mind. I knew we could never really be friends. I had to tell her that I thought it would be best to stick with my policy of not socializing with clients.*

Socialize with the Client, but Keep Your Professional Role

Sometimes it's not a problem to socialize with clients or ex-clients if practitioners remain aware of their roles and responsibilities.

Vivien Schapera, co-director of Alexander Technique of Cincinnati, says that although she does not initiate social invitations with clients, she does sometimes accept them. She has wise advice about socializing with clients and former clients:

➤ *We can be social, but we can't show what I call our "lower selves." We can't show our pettiness, neediness, jealousies, and so on. We tend to work from our higher selves, so clients tend to think we are better than we really are. We may thrive on this adulation. However, once we become friends with our clients, we may find ourselves resorting to our lower selves in the same way we do in the comfort of our own homes and with our closest friends. If we get into a difficult situation with a friend who is also a client, if they push our buttons, we have to pull ourselves out of being 3 years old, regardless of how justified we might feel. We must remember that we are the practitioners, always. It never goes away. No matter how hard it is, we have to be "big," we have to be the role model, we have to be generous, we have to give the benefit of the doubt, and so on. It's a delicate and fragile thing to have multiple roles. So if we take someone on as both a client and a friend, we are never justified in letting them down.*

Learn How to Turn Down Invitations

Practitioners can feel awkward or unkind when they have to refuse a client's invitation. It's a good idea to assure them that it's part of your professional policy, not a personal rejection. You can say, "Thank you so much for thinking of me; however, I have a policy of never socializing with clients. The relationship we have is special and important for the work that we do together. It would change if we tried to take it outside these walls. I hope that you understand."

Working with Friends and Relatives

There are several reasons why it's not a good idea to work with friends and relatives. Professionals need to work with an objective, nonjudgmental attitude and not have their own agendas for a client. Clients need to be able to focus on themselves and not be aware of our needs. These goals are impossible when we work with people who are involved in our lives in other ways.

Here's an example of having a personal agenda:

➤ *Your friend Bill is very uptight about his job these days. Aside from being concerned about him, you want him to lighten up because he's not fun to be around. When he comes in for a massage, you are highly motivated to help him to relax. Rather than gently coaxing him to let go at his own pace, as you would for any other client, you try to force his muscles to soften. Your haste says, "Hurry up and relax, Bill!" However, it's hard for him to let go because he senses your impatience. It's a frustrating experience for both of you.*

We can also take friends for granted and not give them the same courtesies we give other clients:

➤ *Your friend Heather comes to you as a paying client because she's stressed out. You've got some errands to do before the session, and since it's just Heather, you know you can start late. Also, you haven't seen her for a while, so you use the session time to catch her up on your news. Is that fair to Heather?*

Working with people we know can be hard on practitioners, too. Friends and family don't always appreciate the amount of time, energy, and money we've put into learning a skill that's now intended to support us. They may think that what they're receiving is just a friendly back rub. Also, friends often don't give us the

Boundary Lessons

While I was attending massage school, I was required to do 50 massages outside of class and document them, so naturally I called on friends and family to be the recipients, and I did not charge them anything, as it is against the law in our state for students to receive any compensation, including a tip. Unfortunately, I found that the friends who had willingly gotten free massage when I was practicing never came to me as a client after I had my license and started charging for massage, which made me feel resentful. I found that my family members expected me to give them a discount just because they were family. It seemed like nobody had respect for my work just because I had prior relationships with them. It made me wish I had offered my practice massages to total strangers instead of friends and family.

> I don't massage my own mother, unless she's in great pain and it's some dire emergency (and no, she doesn't pay, I gladly pay one of my staff members to massage her). The fact is that if I am her therapist, she spends the session filling me in on the family gossip—who's getting married/divorced/going on a trip/got fired from their job, or whatever it is. When she's with another therapist, she settles down and relaxes, and gets much more benefit out of the work than she would if she was with me. I'd prefer to skip the family gossip while I'm working, and she gets the bodywork she really needs. That's sometimes the danger in massaging family members or friends; the focus ends up being somewhere other than the massage.

respect we deserve or take the work as seriously as they would with someone they don't know. They may show up late, not call to cancel, or, especially if we work at home, want to hang around after their sessions.

Occasionally, we can make exceptions, but not often. We can sometimes see a friend or family member on a one-time or occasional basis and not have problems, but we have to give serious consideration to whether we want to work with them regularly.

Mixing Social Occasions with Work

Just as we don't want sessions to be about socializing, social gatherings aren't an appropriate place to display our professional talents. Even students who don't charge for their work shouldn't comply with requests to rub a sore shoulder outside of an office or a workspace. (An exception can be made for students who get together after school to socialize. The social occasions discussed here are those with prospective clients.) It sets a bad precedent to work during our off-hours.

It can be difficult to turn down friends who want free samples like a little back rub, but we can just smile and say, "I'm off duty." Friends and family need to know that it's unfair to ask us to be available during our off-hours for even a shoulder rub. Also, we can tell them that we don't usually take family or close friends as clients, and if they want a professional massage, we can refer them to someone else. The same applies for consulting at a party about someone's bad back. It's tempting to want to show off or sell our work in a social gathering, but it's not an appropriate place for a professional consultation. We can simply give out our business card and ask the person to call during business hours. We can say, "I'd really like to discuss it with you, but I can't really do you justice in an atmosphere like this. How about calling me on Monday, and I'll be glad to talk with you more."

People may be drinking at a social occasion, and that's all the more reason not to do massage at a party or other social situations where people are consuming alcohol. People are less inhibited when they're drinking, and may be more inclined to make an inappropriate remark about massage, to flirt, or to act in other ways that may make it uncomfortable for you to consider them as a future client.

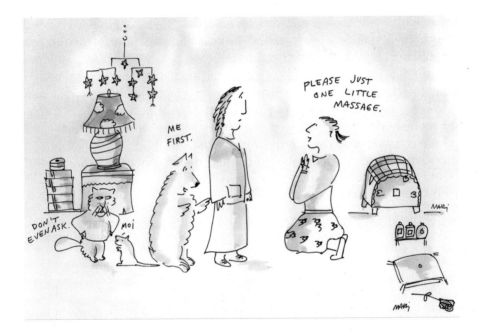

The Complications of Trades and Bartering

Trades and bartering used to be seen as a charming hippie sort of thing, a way to bypass the supposed crassness of money, a way to live more simply. Some people still feel that way about bartering and trading services and goods. However, trading and bartering have the potential for being real pains in the neck and sources of misunderstanding, especially if they are ongoing rather than one-time practices. Many of the practitioners I interviewed have discontinued doing trades or barters. This is an issue primarily for those in private practice, who have the freedom to make their own financial arrangements.

Trading and bartering are problematic because, along with having the potential confusion of changing roles, they lack the clarity and simplicity of a money exchange. We have to work harder to be sure that each side is happy with what is received and each feels the exchange to be balanced. Here's an example:

> *Mary agrees to an ongoing trade of massage with her colleague Donna, but as the exchange progresses, Mary feels less and less satisfied. Although Mary treats Donna as she would a regular client, Donna doesn't do the same. She's never on time, she interrupts the massage to take phone calls, and she seems halfhearted in her efforts.*

In general, trading for bodywork or massage is more likely to be a problem than bartering, when we exchange our work for a tangible object or a service other than bodywork. The intimacy of our work and the possibilities of transference and countertransference can make trading sessions more difficult. When we trade bodywork, each person finds out about the other's physical and sometimes personal problems. That can interfere with how the person who is the client experiences the massage. For instance, if you know that your practitioner has a persistent wrist problem, would you ask her to go deeper? If you know that she's upset over her divorce, would you complain if she were late for your massage?

Here are some ways to minimize the confusion when doing trades and bartering:

Do Only One-Time Trades

Trades have a better chance of working if they are one-time-only practices and not ongoing. For instance, many practitioners who are new in a community trade as a way to introduce their work to other practitioners.

Be Clear About the Details of the Trade from the Beginning

The challenge with trades is to be very clear what the exchange is. It is best to write it down for both parties to see. Some practitioners say they don't like doing trades because they often end up trading one of their $70 sessions for someone else's $50 session. You can trade two sessions for one or one and a half sessions for one, but the point is to enter into the exchange knowing exactly what the trade is and that both parties are satisfied with it.

CONSIDER THIS

If you charge less than a therapist you do a trade with, how would you feel at the conclusion if she says "That will be $20, since I charge more than you do?" You might be shocked that she doesn't consider an hour of your time and skill equal to an hour of her time and skill. Be sure that the expectations of both parties involved are very clear.

Be Careful if You Barter for a Service Rather Than for Something Tangible

Some forms of barter are unprofessional. For example, bartering for psychotherapy isn't generally considered legitimate in the professional psychotherapy community. But what about bartering for other services? One of the difficulties is in being precise. Suppose you're bartering a session for 2 hours of house cleaning. The client's idea of how a house should look after 2 hours of cleaning can be different from yours. If it's not as tidy as you want, then it's awkward to switch from the nonjudgmental practitioner's role to that of the complaining customer. It's also less than desirable for a client to have such an intimate glimpse of your private life and personal habits. A colleague says, "I don't want clients to see what's inside my car—all the clutter and mess—much less what's inside my house." Another colleague says "I was bartering with my hairdresser. Then she used a new perm solution on my hair and I wound up looking like I had stuck my finger in a light socket—not the look I was going for. She assured me it would 'calm down' in a few days, but I was very unhappy with the way it looked, and she wasn't happy when I broke off the trade."

However, it can work to barter for other services that have a set fee and are not highly personal, such as bartering for yoga classes.

Be Clear About Value When Bartering for Goods

The happiest exchanges can be for various goods, particularly artwork. It's important that the value of the item be clear and agreed on by both parties beforehand. Also, if you're bartering for something you haven't seen, you may want to decide what will happen if you don't like the finished product.

REAL EXPERIENCE

When I opened my own business, I bartered with a local artist for some very nice paintings for my office. I couldn't have afforded to buy them outright, and she referred to herself as a "starving artist" who could not have afforded to get regular massage. It was a win-win for both of us. I also bartered with a woman who made a beautiful quilt to cover my massage table. I have a personal policy of not bartering for services, only for goods, and only when I've actually seen the goods the person is offering. I've heard too many horror stories about therapists bartering with other people for and being unhappy with what the end result is, so I just decided from the outset not to do that.

—M.M., LMT

Spell Out How to Terminate the Agreement

Be clear ahead of time about what will happen if one of the parties decides to quit before the exchange is even. Suppose a practitioner is bartering massage for guitar lessons. She's given $200 worth of massage sessions and has received only $100 worth of guitar lessons. At that point, she decides she doesn't really want to practice, and doesn't want any more lessons.

Because they hadn't already resolved how to handle this possibility, they now have some potentially sticky questions to resolve. Since she is the one who changed her mind, does the guitar teacher owe her anything? And if he does owe her the $100 balance, does he have to pay it all immediately? The details can vary, but it's best to work them out ahead of time. Putting them in writing makes clear that you both understand the terms.

If Possible, Trade or Barter with Professionals

It's easiest to trade with someone who is a professional at whatever the service or work is. Professionals usually have a clear idea of their prices and know how to work with clients. In the earlier story about the therapist who was unsatisfied with the wallpaper job in her living room, she would likely have been okay with the trade if the client she had bartered with had worked at the wallpaper store for years and been a professional who was experienced at hanging wallpaper. If you need a professional service, that's probably going to work out much better if you get a professional to do it, whether it's cash or trade.

Be Willing to Say No

Don't agree to a trade or barter just to please the other person, and don't barter for something you don't want or need.

Don't agree to a trade or barter just to please the other person, and don't barter for something you don't want or need.

These situations are unbalanced from the start and can breed resentment. You should also be careful about how many such exchanges you take on at once so that you are not working all week and ending up with no cash. Remember that trades and barters can take more energy than regular clients because of the time spent on negotiating terms as well as the likelihood of misunderstandings.

Despite all the possible problems, trades sometimes work out well. Some practitioners have established workable trades with colleagues, often those who were fellow students, in which the trade feels mutually beneficial and the two give each other valuable feedback.

Other Relationships

Clients that we have other relationships with can sometimes be problematic. So can clients that we've never even met—but have some knowledge of. For example, your friend suffered through a very painful divorce after her husband left her for another woman. What if the "other woman" calls for an appointment? Could you treat her like any other client? What about the parent of the child that you feel bullies your son at school? Or the client who turns out to be the brother of the neighbor that you don't get along with? It can be a challenge to leave our prejudices out of the treatment room. If you don't feel you can, it's best to turn that client over to someone else.

Business Relationships

The ethics of selling products to clients or involving them in business deals is covered in more detail in Chapter 5. To review, there are two main problems:

1. Because of transference, the client may not be as free as a nonclient to refuse to buy whatever the practitioner is selling. Even just a suggestion from a respected or beloved practitioner can feel like an offer the client can't refuse.

2. If something goes wrong—the lotion is messy, the stocks drop, the pillow doesn't seem to help the neck pain—the client may not feel as free as a nonclient to complain or ask for a refund. And you could lose a client if a business deal or product doesn't pan out.

Some spas strongly urge or require their massage therapists to push clients to buy products from the spa. As discussed in Chapter 5, you want to check out a spa's policy on selling to clients and decide whether you are comfortable with it before you commit to the job.

Involving clients in other business transactions can cause resentment, lower the client's respect for the practitioner, and interfere with the therapeutic relationship.

Just as we don't want to engage clients in business, we want to be careful about taking on business associates as clients. Here's the kind of confusion that can happen:

➤ *A massage therapist who is a part-time operating room nurse gave a massage to one of her nursing colleagues. During the massage, when the colleague talked about problems she was having at home and cried, the therapist was appropriately sympathetic and understanding. After that, the colleague started slacking off at work. She excused herself for not doing her part by saying to the nurse/ massage therapist, "I know you understand what a hard time I'm having these days."*

Practitioners also report having problems when they work with someone who is their boss or has authority over them in another setting. For instance, sometimes bosses want to continue acting as if they are in charge when they become clients.

They can be demanding clients, expecting to be given extra time or special concessions. Setting limits with the boss or even contemplating having to set limits can be uncomfortable.

Also, sometimes practitioners rightfully do not wish to know the people for whom they work that intimately, or are afraid the boss might make an inappropriate comment or sexualize the situation.

Minimizing Problems

It's often hard to avoid dual relationships. Sometimes we have good reason to take on a friend as a client, do a trade, barter, or even socialize with a client or an ex-client. For example, we may be the only one in town who practices a particular kind of bodywork, and we think a friend would greatly benefit from that method. We may be the only massage therapist that a shy friend would be comfortable seeing. We may live and work in a small community in which it's hard to avoid social contact with our clients.

When are dual relationships likely to lead to trouble, and when might they work? How can we manage dual relationships with the least stress to clients and to ourselves?

Dual Relationships to Avoid

There are a number of circumstances in which a dual relationship would be likely to lead to problems or be harmful to the client.

Working with Friends or Relatives Who Are in Physical or Emotional Crisis or Actively Dealing with Abuse Issues

The likelihood of intense transference or dependency when a friend or relative is dealing with deep emotional issues makes it difficult to work well with that person. Also, we generally have too much investment in such people to have the objectivity to be helpful. A colleague reports:

> ➤ *My friend had a chronic back problem that flared up right before a vacation. I really wanted to help her. In spite of my best efforts, after an hour she was still in a good deal of pain. Had she been a regular client, I would have been concerned, but I probably would have been able to be more objective. I would have stopped at the end of an hour, knowing that I had done my best and that there may be other factors involved, such as emotional issues. But since it was my friend, I kept trying, which only seemed to make things worse. The fact that I couldn't help her was hard on our friendship, and it took a while for us to be able to talk honestly about what happened.*

Doing Emotionally Oriented or Psychologically Oriented Bodywork

Practitioners of emotionally or psychologically oriented bodywork should avoid dual relationships. These practitioners are always working with deep transference issues and cannot risk the complications that would arise from dual relationships. As with other dual relationships, people who do emotionally-oriented work cannot become friends with clients and can rarely become friends with ex-clients. And it always bears repeating: being trained in such modalities does not make you a psychologist.

Having Sexual Relationships with Clients

As discussed in Chapter 7, maintaining ethical boundaries means that sexual relationships with clients are forbidden and those with ex-clients are entered into with caution and care.

Bringing Clients into Outside Business Deals

As discussed in Chapter 5, involving clients or ex-clients in another business relationship, verges on being unethical.

Tips for Working with Dual Relationships

If you decide to have a dual relationship with a client, here are suggestions for making it less of a problem:

Discuss Your Misgivings with the Prospective Client

If friends or family members want to work with you, talk with them about the problems with changing roles. Let them know they would probably benefit more from going to a practitioner they don't know. If you both still want to proceed, check in with them regularly to make sure no problems are arising.

Keep Your Usual Boundaries and Framework Standards

Because you're already bending boundaries by working with someone you know in another way, you need to be more aware of all other boundaries and framework, not less. You may be tempted to think, "Oh, it's just Bob. I can still be eating my sandwich when he arrives." That would give Bob a message that the setting is not quite professional or safe for him. Aside from interfering with his ability to relax, it's bad advertising for you. Every client is a potential source of referrals; if someone asks Bob how he liked his massage, you want him to endorse you with enthusiasm rather than think, "I hope she acts more like a professional when she's with other clients."

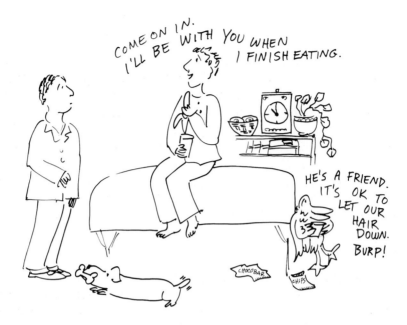

Keep Confidentiality and Session Boundaries

Assure clients with whom you have another relationship that what they say and do inside a session will be held in confidence. Let them know that it's best for the two of you to keep work-related questions and comments inside the office space.

Separate Social Time and Professional Time

Advise clients that they will get more out of their sessions if you don't mix session time with either social or business time—if you don't chitchat during sessions, talk about business, or go to lunch together right before or after sessions. You might want to stop seeing a friend socially while he or she is a client or, at the very least, not take the friendship to another level. If someone is, for instance, a friend that you see socially every few months, you don't want to start having lunch once a week during your work together.

Special Considerations for Students

It's particularly common for students to work with friends and relatives while they are learning their trade. Although this is not usually a good idea for a professional practice, this can be a useful way for students to acquire experience, become accustomed to doing a certain number of sessions a week, and practice their "tableside manner."

Even in a practice situation, the problems of dual relationships arise. Massage students who haven't yet had a lot of experience may be stressed over things that

CONSIDER THIS

We all have a life outside work, and we're all entitled to have fun, but we may still need to be on guard. What if you're in a club with some girlfriends, having a few drinks and celebrating your pal's birthday, and a client you've seen several times professionally comes up and asks you to dance? You don't want to appear rude in refusing—but it's probably for the best if you do refuse. You're drinking, the lights are down low, the music is playing, and you're wearing a sexy outfit. It may be tempting to forget that you are this person's massage therapist and just be a woman out for a night on the town—but you have to consider how that might affect your future professional encounters with this person.

might seem more ordinary to them a few years into their practice, like the friend or family member who shows up late for their massage. One therapist said "My Aunt Marge is chronically late for everything. Everyone in the family jokes that she'll be late for her own funeral. Since I know that, when she says she's coming at 2 p.m., I put that appointment in the book for 2:15 p.m., because I know she isn't going to get there until then. But when I was working in the student clinic, it really stressed me out the day she had an appointment there and showed up late. I felt like the clinic supervisor was waiting to see how I handled it, and I was nervous about it." The same "little things" that come up for students also come up for more experienced professionals when they have dual relationships—keeping a friend's massage from becoming a social occasion, dealing with friends who forget their appointment, expect a free foot massage, and so forth. However, these situations are more common and troublesome for students who are starting their practices and may feel insecure about claiming a professional role and setting appropriate boundaries.

Here are some suggestions to help students start out on the right foot:

Set Boundaries from the Beginning

When you begin to do practice sessions with friends and family, let them know what to expect from the beginning. You can say, for instance, "I appreciate your being a guinea pig now as I'm learning my trade, and the session will be free. When I've graduated and gotten my license, I'll charge all my clients $60" (or whatever amount you plan to charge).

It's easier to set limits at the time the initial appointment is arranged, not after resentment has built because a friend has stayed for 2 hours after her massage. "I'll have an hour available from 2 to 3 o'clock, and then I'll have to take care of some other business." This is often an issue for therapists who work from home;

It's up to you to let friends and family know the boundaries. They may not realize that they're taking advantage of you.

sometimes family and friends don't realize that working at home is still working! You may need to make it clear to those in your circle, if you're working in a home office, that you're seeing clients throughout the day and can't handle drop-in visitors or stay on the phone to chat. It's up to you to let friends and family know the boundaries. They may not realize that they're taking advantage of you.

Treat Free Sessions As if They Were "Real" Sessions: Practice Boundaries

A good way to develop professionalism and help the boundaries stay clear is to treat each session as if the client were paying. Let friends and family members know that they will be treated as regular clients and explain what that means: you want to start and end on time, you'll use appropriate draping, and they may talk if they want, but you won't respond by chatting in the way that you would in a social situation. You can explain that this framework is helpful to you as a student and will also help them get the most out of their sessions. An added bonus is that friends and family members will have the experience of seeing how professional you've become and will be more inspired to recommend you to someone else.

Be Wary of Dual Relationships

Sometimes we're lucky and squeak by without problems with a dual relationship. Usually, though, these relationships lead to anything from minor annoyances (putting extra energy into sorting out misunderstandings) to major problems (being in hot water for unethical behavior). Clients who are entangled in dual relationships with us often don't benefit from our work as much as other clients do. There just isn't the same amount of attention and therapeutic focus.

Decisions about whether to take on a person as a client need to be based on solid professional judgment, not ease and convenience. However despite the drawbacks, dual relationships will probably always be with us. It helps if we realize the problems intrinsic to their nature and take extra precautions to make the professional relationship safe for both parties.

Questions for Reflection

1. Outside of massage or bodywork, have you ever been part of a dual relationship with a friend or family member? How did it work out? If it worked out well, what do you think made it successful? If not, what got in the way?

2. Have you ever been part of a trade? Were you satisfied with what you received from it? If not, what would have made it better?

3. Have you ever been in a situation with a professional or a businessperson in which there was a dual relationship? Were there any problems related to the dual relationship? If not, what do you think helped? If there were problems, what would have helped lessen or eliminate them?

4. At a social occasion, have you ever gotten involved in essentially giving a free consultation or sample of your work to a potential client? How did that work out? If it worked out well, what made the difference? If not, what would you do differently to avoid problems next time?

5. Have you ever gone from being a client to being a friend of a professional of any kind? Were there any issues to work out—for instance, were you disappointed when you found out more about the professional? If it has worked out well to be a friend, do you think that it would always work out well to become a friend of the professionals in your life? Why or why not? If it didn't work out well, what made the difference?

---

thePoint® To learn more about the concepts discussed in this chapter, visit http://thePoint .lww.com/Allen-McIntosh4e

CHAPTER *11*

Boundaries and the Internet

Although the preceding chapters have addressed matters pertaining to the Internet, these lessons have to be reinforced. The Internet has had a profound impact on our lives, both personal and business. The boundary lines have gotten blurred—and sometimes seem to have disappeared altogether. Our actions on the Internet have the potential to violate the code of ethics, our clients' boundaries, and harm our own reputations. Extra diligence is required in order to protect our clients and protect ourselves.

Many people are used to using the Internet for multiple purposes: school, work, e-mail, banking, and bill-paying, social media, blogging, advertising, research, shopping, just to name a few.

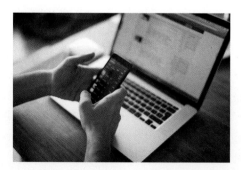

Smart phones, tablets, and notebooks have made it possible to stay tethered to the Internet no matter where you are. The propensity of some people to take pictures and videos—and share those on the Internet—has almost made it a law of the universe that we should all assume that anything we say or do might wind up posted on the Internet.

Client Privacy

Every contact with a client, from the first phone call to the last visit, is subject to our obligation to keep their information confidential. That means their records, whether handwritten or electronic, anything that they communicate to you verbally (or nonverbally, as is sometimes the case due to the nature of our work), and just the fact that they are our clients at all, is confidential information and must be treated as such.

Not only is the rule of confidentiality a part of the code of ethics; it is also the law in regulated states, and it can also go as far back as our mandate to first do no harm. Although people tend to think of that in terms of not causing physical harm to the client, such as ignoring contraindications for massage, it can also mean any kind of harm, such as sharing information that is supposed to be kept private, deriding clients in public (even when you don't mention their name—more about that later), or doing anything that violates the sanctity of the therapeutic relationship.

HIPAA

HIPAA, the Health Insurance Portability Accountability Act, was created in 1996 to protect the privacy of the client when information is electronically transmitted. In theory, this is meant to protect the individual's identifying information and personal data when health records are transmitted between health plans, health plan clearinghouses, and health-care providers who use electronic means of communication. In reality, it goes deeper than that. Massage therapists are technically not considered health-care providers under the statutes in the majority of regulated states. That does not excuse us from following the spirit of the privacy rules of HIPAA, which serve numerous purposes:

- Gives patients more control over their health information
- Sets boundaries on the use and release of health records
- Establishes appropriate safeguards that the majority of health-care providers and others must achieve to protect the privacy of health information
- Holds violators accountable with civil and criminal penalties that can be imposed if they violate patients' privacy rights
- Strikes a balance when public health responsibilities support disclosure of certain forms of data
- Enables patients to make informed choices based on how individual health information may be used
- Enables patients to find out how their information may be used and what disclosures of their information have been made

CONSIDER THIS

If you use a computer in your lobby/waiting area, be sure that any client who is waiting is not seeing any client information. Never leave your online scheduler, e-mail, client database, or other things that may contain client names and information open on the screen where anyone may see it. It's easy to get distracted when clients are waiting, so set your screensaver to go dark very quickly when it's out of use so that you won't forget about it.

- Generally limits release of information to the minimum reasonably needed for the purpose of the disclosure
- Generally gives patients the right to obtain a copy of their own health records and request corrections
- Empowers individuals to control certain uses and disclosures of their health information (Source: Center for Disease Control: HIPAA Privacy Rule and Public Health, Guidance from the CDC and the U.S. Department of Health and Human Services, accessible online at http://www.cdc.gov/mmwr/preview/mmwrhtml/m2e411a1.htm

Therapists who work in chiropractic offices, hospitals, hospice care, or other medical settings may have more knowledge of HIPAA than others. Even for those working alone in other settings, there are some insurance policies that do cover massage, as well as opportunities to work with personal injury and worker's compensation cases. The fact that we may not be involved in accepting insurance does not mean that we shouldn't be familiar with what the privacy rules are intended to accomplish—to protect the privacy of anyone seeking services. Many of us consider ourselves members of the health-care team, even when the law does not consider us as such. Many of us have referral relationships with doctors and other health-care providers; whether that is the case or not, we're under an obligation to safeguard the client's privacy as if we were guarding all the gold in Fort Knox.

Any electronic service you are using, such as online booking for clients, or transmitting any of their information, even if it's nothing more than their name and address, should be done over secure sites.

From a technical standpoint, any client information should only be transmitted securely. If you're not technically savvy, educate yourself or hire a computer expert to help you understand the ins and outs of secure transmission. For example, "http" preceding a website means that it is not a secure site. "Https" indicates that it is. Banks, credit card companies, health-care entities, any site that you are conducting commerce with, such as buying something over

CONSIDER THIS

You might be a therapist who doesn't particularly consider yourself a health-care provider, nor have any ambition to be considered one. However, let's say that a long-time client is involved in a car accident, and her attorney sends you a signed release to obtain the records of the care she has received from you during a certain period of time. (a) You're going to appear totally unprofessional if you're one of those therapists who doesn't keep records and (b) You can't just dash that response off in a quick e-mail without being sure it is being securely transmitted. If you still use a fax machine that is being transmitted over a land line, you can find out from your phone service provider whether or not that is a secure line. If it isn't, you shouldn't be transmitting any client identifying information or health care records over it. The same goes for your Internet connection.

the Internet and giving your credit card information, should have the "https" designation. In a nutshell, "https" means that a web page is utilizing a form of encryption known as a Secure Socket Layer. While it is safer than http, there are plenty of creative hackers out there who can get around that, as evidenced by people hacking into banks, the Social Security Administration, and the Pentagon. Still, it does offer an additional layer of protection. Any electronic service you are using, such as on-line booking for clients, or transmitting any of their information, even if it's nothing more than their name and address, should be done over secure sites.

Phones and Texting

The use of your phone in any capacity, answering calls or texting while you are with a client, is an absolute violation of your client's time and goodwill. I've seen complaints posted on social media from consumers of massage who stated that they noticed their therapist only had one hand on them and found that they were texting! The client is paying for your time and attention. That means your time and attention should be devoted to them, and no one else.

Texting your spouse (in the lobby, not in the treatment room with the client present) to say you'll be late is fine. Texting your spouse to say "Mary Hill decided to get a 90 minute appointment instead of an hour, so I'll be late getting home," is not—even if your spouse knows Mary Hill as well as you do. You simply do not name your clients, in conversation, texting, or any other communications, other than to those health-care providers, emergency contact, attorney or others that they have given you a signed release to do so.

One of my favorite apps is a posture analysis app. It involves taking pictures of the clients, which of course will only be done with their permission. Massage therapists sometimes forget that confidentiality should be honored even when communicating with a colleague or peer. In a group practice, spa, or franchise situation, it should be made clear to the client that they may be seen by more than one therapist and that everyone employed there may see their records. But let's say you're eating lunch with a massage therapist friend who practices across town, and you start telling her how cool the posture app is, and whip out your phone to show her. It would be an ethics violation if you showed the client's pictures to someone who is not directly involved in his or her care.

E-mail

You may desire to have a client's e-mail address for several reasons. Perhaps you send out a monthly newsletter, or announcements of specials you're offering. If that's the case, you should be following the rules of secure and private e-mail communications.

Using an Internet mail service, such as MailChimp or Constant Contact is the best way to avoid making a mistake that could result in a privacy violation, such as your clients seeing each other's e-mail addresses. That may sound like a simple thing, but it is not. Many people use their name as their address, like lauraallen@website.com. When you consider that we are not even supposed to tell anyone the names of our clients, sending out an e-mail and failing to use the BCC (blind carbon copy) feature could result in everyone seeing the names and e-mail addresses of other people. It's an easy mistake to make, and I've had it happen to me in communications from other business people who ought to know better.

E-mailing clients should not be done without their express permission. I have a line on my own intake form that asks for the e-mail address with the statement *if you would like to receive our monthly newsletter and special announcements.* Another line asks clients if they would like to receive e-mail, calls, or text reminders of their appointment times. If you are using an online scheduler, those will state on the scheduler that it will automatically send e-mail appointment reminders to clients or give them the option of receiving a text.

Every e-mail you send to a client should give them the option to unsubscribe from receiving e-mail from you. Lack of an unsubscribe option is characteristic of spam. Even if you have permission to add the client to your e-mail list, avoid slamming people with e-mail, or you'll lose subscribers. Your clients don't need to hear

---

Boundary Lessons

Don't take it personally whenever a client declines to give you his or her e-mail address. Some people don't use e-mail at all; while some people may find that incredible, you have to remember that not everyone uses the Internet. Some people depend on the phone, texts, and instant messaging instead of e-mail. People may have their own reasons for not giving out their e-mail address. Perhaps, they feel like they already have too much e-mail to wade through on a daily basis. Or they may share an e-mail address with a spouse or other family members and don't want that person to know they're seeing you. I used to feel a little upset and disappointed when people didn't provide their e-mail address on the intake form. I felt insulted that they didn't want to get my newsletter or hear about my specials. I was complaining about it one day to another therapist friend of mine, and she said "You have to remember it's not all about *you*. It's about what the client feels comfortable with, and we have to respect that." She's right, and I've never taken it personally again.

—S.L., MT

---

from you on a daily basis. Use your e-mail wisely and in a professional manner. Avoid sending nonbusiness-related e-mails to your client list, They provided it to you on the premise that they would be receiving e-mail related to the business, not jokes or recipes from the Internet.

Social Media

Social media is fun, isn't it? People who use it may reconnect with people they haven't seen since grade school, find long-lost relatives, meet up with other massage therapists or otherwise like-minded people through all the groups and forums, share news, jokes, videos, inspirational posts, rants, and any number of things. Social media is also a great tool for promoting your business, used in the right way.

As I'm writing this, Facebook has over 1.65 billion users. Over 80 million photographs per day are uploaded to Instagram. Twitter has over 320 million active users. Everybody knows everybody else's business! People post their love affairs, their breakups, their opinions, their complaints, their pictures, their politics, their prayers, their porn, their deaths and births, their blessings, and their problems. Social media has made the world a much smaller place. It makes it easy to keep up with friends, family, and followers. It's also, unfortunately, one more opportunity to violate client confidentiality, and another opportunity to harm your own reputation (or have someone else harm it) as a professional massage therapist.

Your clients may not be on your FB page, but mutual friends or family members may be. Let's say you make a post about a client that you thought was rude, or otherwise didn't suit you for some reason. In your anger, you might say "besides being rude, she had the worst case of acne I've ever seen and spent the whole session unloading on me about her divorce and her child being diagnosed with Oppositional Defiant Disorder, and complaining about how he's always in trouble at school." Some local person on your page may instantly know who you're referring to. They may also wonder if you talk about them!

Take Facebook, for example. There are numerous groups for massage therapists on Facebook. I am the administrator of a couple of our state groups and organizational pages myself. As the ones I administer are much smaller than a national or worldwide group, and primarily used to share information such as local continuing education classes or a local therapist selling a massage table, there's not much inappropriate sharing in those groups. Some of the larger, more open groups are a different story entirely. It's routine for therapists to post body-shaming comments about clients who are overweight or have excessive body hair, or some other condition that they can make fun of.

➤ *Can you imagine if you were a person thinking about getting your first massage, and you saw the following social media post:*

I had a client today who must have weighed 300 pounds and I bet she hasn't shaved her legs in years! She looked like a fat grizzly bear! EEEEW!

➤ *Or what about this one:*

Some people just have ugly feet! I got a new client today who had the ugliest feet I've ever seen. He had weird-looking long bony toes and a bunion the size of a golf ball. He wanted me to work on his feet and I really wanted to refuse. Just the thought of touching them made me cringe!

Yes, those are unfortunately real posts from Facebook. First of all, if you are in judgment of people's bodies in that manner, then you have no business being a massage therapist. It's part of the job to be accepting and nonjudgmental of people who are fat, bony, hairy, hairless, white or any other color, people who have stretch marks, scars, warts, bunions, corns, physical deformities, amputations, and any other thing that may be unique to their body. Second, posting such things on social media is a surefire way to scare off anyone who might be thinking about visiting a

CONSIDER THIS

Even if you do not specifically use the celebrity's name, you may still violate confidentiality. Social media posts like "I just massaged the head coach of the Miami Dolphins!" or "The CEO of Verizon just got a massage from me!" are a violation . . . it takes less than 3 seconds to find that person's name on a search engine.

massage therapist and you in particular, if your name is on the post. It makes the whole profession look bad!

There are very few people in the world who don't have some part of their body that they wish were different—including supermodels. How would *you* feel if you were in that client's shoes? What if you visited a dermatologist and later saw a post she made about your bad case of eczema? You wouldn't like it at all. Your doctor is not on social media making posts about your condition—thank goodness—and you are held to the same standard.

Many people have let their desire to brag override the confidentiality rule. I've seen numerous posts like "Guess what! I'm massaging Lady Gaga tonight before her concert and I get to be backstage!" or "I just massaged Tom Brady and he gave me a $100 tip!" It's incredible that any massage therapist doesn't see the wrong in that. If a celebrity gives you a written testimonial, leaves a review on a website, posts on his or her own Twitter account that he or she just got an amazing massage from you, or allows you to take a selfie with him or her while he or she is at your office, then the person knows it's out there for public consumption. Otherwise, it is a serious ethics violation.

Massage therapists sometimes lose sight of the fact that it is not the client who is bound to abide by a code of ethics. It is us!

Otherwise, it's confidential, and all clients should be able to have the expectation of privacy, whether it's the star quarterback or the minister from the church across the street from your office.

Even in the event a client treats you badly, or makes an inappropriate overture, you are still obligated to safeguard his or her confidentiality. It is *not* okay to make a post like this:

Don't take any checks from Betty Smith! She wrote me a check for a gift certificate and it bounced!

or a post like this:

Warning all Lakeland massage therapists, if a client named John Doe calls you for an appointment, refuse it! He is just a pervert!

Your Own Social Media Image

Other than making inappropriate posts about clients on social media, have you considered how you are presenting yourself? If you're identifying yourself as a massage therapist on your social media pages, and posting pictures of yourself holding a shot of tequila in your hand while you're dancing on the bar in a local club, or posting pictures of yourself in revealing clothing and that "come hither" look on your face, how do you think that appears to clients? What message are you trying to send?

You may think you're safe if your privacy settings are set so that only your own friends can see what you post, but that's not really so. Let's say that your neighbor is also a social media friend. He has a few buddies over to watch the football game, and his computer screen is up so everyone in the room can see it. There you are in a picture taken at his last barbecue, when you all got a little too drunk and decided to go skinny dipping in his pool. You didn't even know those pictures were taken.

You can harm your own reputation without even thinking about it. Or maybe you did know, and you were showing off for the camera, not thinking in your alcohol-befuddled state what the consequences might be. His friends see your picture on the screen, ask who that is, and he says "Oh, that's my hot neighbor across the street. She owns a massage business on 4th Avenue." You suddenly find yourself inundated with calls from males who have seen your picture and they want a massage—and more. You can harm your own reputation without even thinking about it.

It's Not All about Sex

If you've allowed clients to be on your personal social media pages, or your privacy settings are on "public," it's not only the sexual component that you need to consider. Everyone has differences of opinion, and people know that. Maybe you don't discuss your politics, your religion, and other personal beliefs with your clients, which is a wise idea. However, let's say you're all hot and bothered about the government, and your social media posts are filled with rants about how you hate the president, or you think all Democrats are morons, or the mayor of your town is an idiot, or you're insulting to any certain population of people. The client you

CONSIDER THIS

Celebrities who might be identifiable, even though you don't name them, are not the only potential violation. Let's say you make a post about a client that you thought was rude, or otherwise didn't suit you for some reason. In your anger, you might say "Besides being rude, she had the worst case of acne I've ever seen and spent the whole session unloading on me about her divorce and her child being diagnosed with Oppositional Defiant Disorder, and complaining about how he's always in trouble at school." Even though the person you made the post about is not on your FB page, some local person on your page may instantly know who you're referring to. They may also wonder if you talk about them!

thought was so nice, and who you thought really liked you, may (understandably) take offense at being lumped in a category of people that you consider morons, and find another massage therapist who isn't so publicly opinionated and insulting to people based on their political beliefs. Especially in a small town, word gets around. That client may be volunteering at Democratic headquarters and say to the other people there, "By the way, that massage therapist down the street thinks Democrats are all a bunch of morons. She's a good therapist but I'm going to find someone else who doesn't make daily Facebook posts about how stupid we all are for supporting the president."

You have just harmed your business standing in your own community by making a comment on social media that may have been harmless if you had said it privately to a friend—but when posting something on the Internet, you should act as if everyone in the world may see it—because in fact, they may.

REAL EXPERIENCE

There is a controversial church located in the small town where I live and practice. Over the years, many people have made accusations that the church is a cult; they've been embroiled in lawsuits, and made the local and national news from time to time. Former church members have made charges of abuse at the hands of leadership and other members; they've had picket lines, and sometimes there have been armed guards outside the church. I had several clients that I didn't even know were members of that church; after all, I don't ask any questions about my clients' religion on my intake form, and as I make it a point not to delve into my clients' private lives or discuss controversial subjects, it never came up in conversation. After our local paper reported a case of a former member suing them, I shared that on my Facebook page and made some derogatory comments about the church and its members—although personally I've never even been there; I was just sharing what had been said in the paper and adding my own opinion about it. The day after I made the post, a client called to cancel her appointment. When I asked if she would like to reschedule it, she said "No, I'm going to have to find another therapist. I heard that you were talking badly about my church online, and I just can't see you again. I'm also going to tell our other church members not to patronize your business." I was shocked. I had no idea that she was a member there, and I had also never considered that anything I said on Facebook could cause me to lose business, but it did. I lost three people on account of it. I now keep my mouth shut about things like that.

—S.H., LMT

Another thing to consider is whether or not you have social media pages for your business.

Facebook abounds with those; I had one for my clinic. If you allow others to post on your page, you're taking the risk that those will all be nice and complimentary, when that may not be the case. Deleting complaints from your page can also backfire—the person may state on their own page that when they made a valid (in their perception) complaint on your page, that you deleted it. Take a lesson from the way major companies respond to consumer complaints online. Usually, it is something along the lines of "We are sorry that you had a bad experience at our company, and we hope that you will give us another chance." Avoid being argumentative, which will make you look even worse, even though there may be a valid excuse for why the customer had a bad experience. Here's an example: "I'm sorry the noise from the road construction in front of our business was a distraction the day you came for your massage. We did not know that was going to be happening, or we would have given you the option to reschedule. We will be glad to offer you a discount for a return visit." That kind of response makes you appear much more responsive and caring to the customer instead of responding in a snippy way, or ignoring their complaint.

Your Own Website

Consumers expect businesses to have a website these days. Unless you are practicing out of your home and are only accepting word-of-mouth referrals, it will help your business to have one. If you belong to one of the professional associations such as AMTA or ABMP, a simple website is part of your membership package. You may build your own site if you have that capability, or hire or barter with a professional for that service. In addition to informing people about your business, your website can actively be an income stream for you, if you offer online gift certificate sales, retail products or act as an affiliate site, have online booking for appointments, or online registration for classes you may be offering. It can be a timesaver for you and convenient for clients if you put a downloadable intake form on your website, allowing people to have it filled out before they arrive for their appointment. Remember, if you are collecting any client information, taking online bookings, asking for credit card numbers or other personal information on your site, you must have a secure website.

Your website should be an honest representation of you, your business, your qualifications, your services and prices, and your policies. It's sometimes shocking to see the way things are misrepresented on the Internet. I once visited a massage school that I had seen a picture of online, and it showed the school at the foot of a mountain, with a big meadow in front, a very beautiful and pastoral setting. I was incredulous when I got there and discovered that the mountain was actually about 30 miles away from the school, and the school had been photoshopped onto the picture at the bottom of the mountain.

Most regulated states require you to have your license number displayed on any advertising, including a website. Be sure that you are in compliance with the requirements in your jurisdiction. You want to highlight your qualifications, so listing any specialty certifications or areas of additional training that you have are a good idea.

Having your services listed on your website will make it clear to the public what you do—and what you do not do. A professional-looking website can make it clear that you are a professional massage therapist, not a sex worker. When a consumer sees "Laura Allen, Clinical Massage Therapist" followed up by a description of the conditions you work with, such as carpal tunnel syndrome, low back pain or the like, that lessens the possibility that you'll get phone calls about providing sexual services.

If your website is unclear about what you do, you may be unwittingly contributing to the number of calls you get for sexual services, or the number of people who act inappropriately once they are already in your office or on the table. Let's say your business name is something like "Blissful Massage" or "Love Your Body Massage." You need to be extra clear on your website and other advertising that you are offering therapeutic massage. A few days ago, a local attorney sent me a solicitation he had received from a sex worker masquerading as a massage therapist. She was actually calling her business "Exquisite Conclusions." One can only assume that she thinks that sounds classier than "Happy Endings." Her blatant solicitation left no doubt about what she was offering, but if the name of your business or your description of it sounds ambiguous, you may be courting trouble.

Having your policies clearly stated on your website can educate the public and offer you a measure of self-protection and something to point to when a client complains—but don't let that be the only place they exist. Some clients may not use the Internet or may have heard of you through another source—and they still need to be informed of your policies. Your policies in regards to late arrivals, cancellations, gift certificates, refunds, and so forth should be detailed not only on your website but also on a sign in your office, on your brochures, or on a separate policy sheet that you give to clients when they visit your office for the first time. Your intake form should have a place for the client to sign stating that they have been informed of your office policies. In the interest of treating everyone fairly and equally, you can't leave clients to guess what your policies are, you can't expect them to adhere to policies they have not been informed of, and you don't need to make them up as you go along.

Online Review Sites

The Internet abounds these days with sites where consumers can leave reviews of businesses. Have you ever looked to see what they're saying about you?

Based on my own searching around these sites, a lot of times, it is not the skill—or lack thereof— of the therapist that gets a bad review. Most complaints are about attitude, lack of listening to the client, not giving them what they paid for and what they expected to get, and other such offenses. Here is an actual review of one business:

➤ *I went to _____ in _____. What a terrible experience. I was given incorrect directions which made me 7 minutes late for a booked, hour and a half appointment. I was informed that I would only be getting an hour and 15 minutes because I was late, but I would be paying for the full hour and one half. I complained that I was late because I was given the wrong directions and was told that's too bad. I wound up getting a 1 hour massage that was poorly performed. She didn't adjust the head rest, she forgot to do my left hand and neck, and knew nothing about how to massage feet. I will NEVER go there again.*

Here's another:

➤ *I bought a package of six gift certificates from _____ at a special price. It did not say anything on the advertisement for the special, or on the gift certificates themselves, that it was for new clients only, and the therapist did not mention that when I made the purchase. Imagine my embarrassment when several of my coworkers, whom I had gifted with the certificates for Christmas, reported to me that they were charged an additional $25 because they had been to the business before. I was mortified and when I called the business, the owner was not apologetic at all. When I told her that wasn't on the advertisement I had seen in the paper, which was what spurred me to buy the gift certificates, nor was it on the certificates, she said "Well, it's on my website, and that's how most people book their appointments." I will never spend another dime at that business.*

We have to remember that one person's perception of a good massage may not match someone else's, but bad reviews can be devastating to a business when there are enough of them. Here's one such review:

➤ *She has absolutely no idea what she's doing; all she did was bathe me in lotion. She rushed through everything; she massaged half of my arms and my legs. That was basically a rub; I wouldn't call it a massage. But at the end, she massaged my shins so hard and for so long that I literally got shin splints. She didn't seem to like the job; it looks like she is just there to collect paychecks. Honestly, she has no business working as a massage therapist; she needs to work somewhere that has zero interaction with people, maybe a bank teller at the drive thru! NO PERSONALITY!*

And another:

➤ *I went to _____ for a massage, and what a rip-off. The massage was mediocre, and the therapist took up about 15 minutes doing some kind of thing where she was just placing her hands on me, not even moving. She told me she was balancing my chakras, whatever that is. They have the price listed as $80 an hour, but when I was checking out, the receptionist informed me that a $20 tip was expected. I told her I wasn't tipping at all and that I wouldn't be back. It rubs me the wrong way, no pun intended, to be held up for a tip when the service wasn't even what I expected. I booked a massage, not some kind of wishy-washy stuff I didn't want to begin with.*

It's next to impossible to get bad reviews removed from these sites. With that thought in mind: *Give people good service.* Treat every massage like it's the best massage you're ever going to give. Give people what they pay for and what they book for—and avoid throwing in things that people have not asked for and unfamiliar with just because it is what *you* want to do. It is not about you; it is about the client. State your financial policies clearly. State your gift certificate policies clearly. If you have a receptionist or others answering the telephone, it's helpful to have a printed list of directions beside the phone (and also on your website) that they can refer to. Have your office policies stated clearly on your website in regards to late arrivals and missed appointments. If you give someone incorrect directions, you shouldn't penalize them for being late. Many of the worst reviews on the Internet are about poor customer service and poor communication. The best action is always preventative action.

The best action is always preventative action.

You can never please all of the people all of the time, but you can be proactive in your practice of massage therapy and the manner in which you conduct your business. We all have off days, and you'll have the occasional complaining client who is having an off day and decides to take it out on you. An occasional complaint does not mean the end of your business, but if a number of bad reviews complain about the same thing, then it's time to take a personal inventory, and recognize that you may indeed have habits or policies that people consider to be poor business practices.

The Good, the Bad, and the Ugly

To summarize this chapter, the Internet can be used for many things—the good, the bad, and the ugly. It's up to you to be diligent in safeguarding client privacy, diligent in not committing any ethical violations on the Internet, and to be diligent in protecting your own online reputation.

Questions for Reflection

1. Think of a situation where you've seen something on the Internet—an unflattering video or photograph of someone—that they were probably unaware was being taken. Imagine that it is you in the photograph or video. How would you feel? Would you feel embarrassed? Would you feel angry at the person who took it and put it on the Internet? How would you deal with it?

2. Look at all the pictures you have posted on your social media sites. If a potential client was looking at those pictures, what kind of impression do you think they would form of you? Do you think they would view you as a professional? Or do you think they may get the wrong idea?

3. If you participate in massage groups on the Internet, go to one of the group pages and spend an hour reading all the posts and comments. Pretend that you are a client who is thinking about getting your first massage. Have a piece of paper to use as a score card. How many posts and comments do you see that would convince you that you should get a massage? How many posts and comments do you see that would convince you that you shouldn't get a massage? Now pretend that you are a physician. How many posts and comments do you see that would make you think "I'd feel good about referring someone to that massage therapist?" How many posts and comments do you see that would make you think "I'd never refer anyone to that massage therapist?" Total those results. How do you think massage therapists are representing themselves overall in the group you just analyzed?

4. Do some Internet research of your own, and visit the websites of other massage therapists. Do you think they are giving the business or individual therapist a professional image? What problems do you see with any of the sites? If you were a member of the public searching for massage, is there something that would make you wonder whether or not the person is offering legitimate massage therapy, or is there something that might give you the impression that they are offering sexual services?

5. Have you ever written a bad review of a business on the Internet? If so, think back on that. Revisit the website where you left the review, and read the other reviews that are there. Are most of them sharing your complaint, or are the majority of reviews complimentary of the business? If that's the case, do you think it is possible that you were personally having a bad day and taking it out on the waitress, the business owner, or other person you were dealing with? Or in retrospect, do you feel that your review was perfectly justified? If you realize that you were personally having a bad day and wanted to delete the review, which may have been unfair to the business, would you attempt to get your review deleted, or decide that's too much trouble and leave it there?

CHAPTER 12

Help with Boundaries: Support, Consultation, and Supervision

Few of us have training in professional relationship skills. True, our common sense and natural instincts are often enough to get us by, but to become solid professionals, we often need outside help and support.

Support can help keep our spark and enthusiasm for our work alive, and that can make a difference in how well we keep boundaries. Learning how to practice good boundaries isn't merely a question of memorizing rules; we can know what we're supposed to do and still make mistakes. How well we maintain boundaries can depend on our overall emotional health and even on how we're feeling on any particular day. Discouragement, loneliness, and boredom take their toll on boundary skills. Perhaps the reason for the most common boundary problem—practitioners using clients as a captive audience—comes from the fact that many practitioners feel isolated and want someone to talk with.

Nobody tells us this in school, but it can be lonely out there. Some of us work in isolation—in our homes, in a private office— and we're alone with clients who may be needy or hurting and looking to us for relief. Even if we work in a spa or an office with other massage therapists, we may not receive enough support in our everyday work lives.

Nobody tells us this in school, but it can be lonely out there.

Most practitioners find that this work isn't as simple as just giving a massage. We work every day with issues of intimacy, dependency, and pain. We all have unresolved beliefs and attitudes that can get in our way. For instance, some of us were raised to believe that we shouldn't complain about aches and pains, that suffering in silence shows strength. How will we feel about clients who come in with a long list of complaints—as is their right? Some of us were brought up to feel that taking care of ourselves and saying no to others is selfish. Will we then be able to draw the line when a client with a sore back wants an appointment on our day off?

Consultation:
A meeting with a professional trained in psychological dynamics to get advice about and insight into a particular client or issue.

Supervision:
An ongoing arrangement made with a professional trained in psychological dynamics for help with the relationship aspects of a practitioner's work.

Regardless of our work setting, how well we handle the relationship aspect of our work can make or break our practices. We need to build into our work lives an abundance of ways to get support, feedback, and new perspective.

Several options for help are available: **consultation**; clinical **supervision**, both in groups and individually; peer support groups; peer supervision groups; and mentoring. Since most of these are still new ideas for the profession, this chapter explores them in detail.

Basics of Consultation, Supervision, and Groups

Many practitioners are learning how to untangle client relationships by consulting with another professional. This might be a one-time consultation about a perplexing situation or ongoing supervision for support and insight.

The consultant or supervisor should be someone who is both experienced in psychological dynamics and appreciative of the issues involved in bodywork and massage therapy. That would be either a bodyworker or massage therapist who also has training or credentials in relationship dynamics or a mental health practitioner who respects the special problems associated with bodywork and massage therapy. The mental health practitioner doesn't need to be trained in bodywork or massage techniques, since technique won't be discussed (see "Choosing a Consultant or Supervisor" later in this chapter).

Consultation

In a consultation, you and your consultant meet outside the session to discuss a particular client or situation. Although the professional might be a psychotherapist or counselor, this kind of consultation isn't the same as psychotherapy. The purpose is to deal with work-related issues. Although you might discover your countertransference issues, personal subjects won't be probed to the same depth as they would be in psychotherapy. Here are some examples of how a consultant could help:

➤ *Massage therapist Mary dreads the days when she sees her client Fred, who constantly complains about his life. Try as she might to be patient, Mary always ends up feeling irritated by his negative outlook.*

In this case, a consultant might, for instance, help Mary realize that Fred reminds her of her father, who disappointed her with his sour outlook on life. Simply having an awareness of how she might be transferring feelings about her father to her client could help Mary work with the client more objectively and compassionately. (If this were psychotherapy, Mary would probably be urged to explore her history and feelings about her father in greater depth.) Also, having that insight would probably help Mary to respond more positively when other clients turn out to be complainers.

➤ *Bodyworker Bob has a client who sometimes cries about her failing marriage during her sessions. Lately, she has seemed more depressed, crying frequently and saying she feels hopeless. Bob wants the client to feel free to express her emotions with him, but he has never been entirely comfortable with her crying, and he now feels overwhelmed by her despair. He thinks she should see a counselor but doesn't know how to suggest that without hurting her feelings or making her feel rejected.*

Bob could discuss several issues with a consultant. He may want to explore his discomfort when a client cries. He might learn, for instance, that crying is generally a healthy release for clients and that he doesn't need to be concerned about occasional tears or feel that he must cheer up the client. He may also learn that in this case, the client could be showing signs of the kind of depression that needs expert help. A consultant could help him identify those warning signals. Furthermore, Bob could learn some skills in referring a client to a counselor. In this instance, he could let her know that although he is concerned and committed to working with her as her massage therapist, he also wonders if she might want to seek professional counseling to help her get through this difficult time.

When to Use Consultation

Here are some red flags that could indicate you would benefit from a consultation:

- Any strong negative feelings about a client that persist, such as frequently feeling impatient or annoyed with a client, feeling drained by a client, or downright disliking a client
- Strong positive feelings about a client, wanting to make special exceptions for a client without objective reasons, or wanting to have a sexual relationship with a client
- Working with a client who is actively dealing with issues of sexual or physical abuse
- Working with a client who seems unusually depressed or who you suspect might be mentally unbalanced
- Having trouble setting limits with a particular client

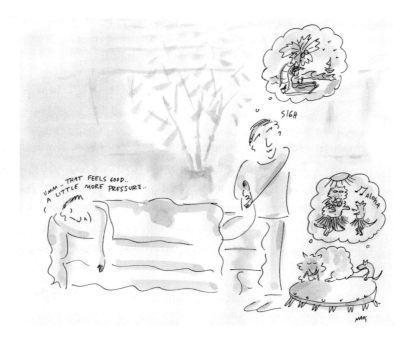

Supervision

Rather than waiting until they have a problem with a client or are in trouble, many practitioners choose ongoing supervision to gain new awareness and ease in their relationships with clients and to break the isolation of their practices. Supervision can also help when you feel bored with your work. Again, this type of supervision is not about the hands-on aspect of your work; it's about helping you improve your professional relationships with clients.

"Supervision" may sound like someone telling you what to do or how to run your business, and that may make you wary. However, a good supervisor supports and guides rather than giving unasked-for advice or making you feel inadequate. Time with a supervisor should feel like a visit with a helpful, friendly teacher.

Unlike a consultation, which is generally a one-time or occasional meeting, with supervision, you would get together on a regular basis, perhaps monthly. The goal is to increase your awareness of yourself as a professional and to clarify your strengths and vulnerabilities in the relationship aspect of dealing with clients.

Good supervision can give you confidence and free you up to do your best work.

(Getting a consultation is a good way to check out how well you would work with another professional you are considering for a supervisor.)

Supervision could make your work life more satisfying by helping you understand stumbling blocks that get in your way and by giving you support when you need it, for instance, with setting limits, trusting your intuition, or appreciating your assets. Good supervision can give you confidence and free you up to do your best work.

A colleague reports:

➤ *At first, I didn't like the idea of supervision, mostly because I was afraid I'd look stupid. After all, I'd been practicing for many years, and I thought I was supposed to have all the answers. However, a friend seemed to be getting so much from her supervision that I decided to try it. To my delight, it was a big boon to my practice. My attitude and behavior toward my clients became more understanding, and clients responded positively to that. The client I had thought was annoying and demanding turned out to be a likable woman who was just frightened about giving up control. The client that I had judged as weird and eccentric turned into a loyal long-term client when I became less judgmental of him. I began to understand my unhelpful patterns and also how to help clients feel more comfortable with me as their practitioner. My practice increased and I am happier with my work life.*

When to Use Supervision

You don't need a special reason to seek out supervision. You may just want to grow as a professional, or you may want your practice to be more satisfying. While you would seek out a one-time consultation for a particular client, for instance, you can use supervision when you notice patterns that don't serve you well in your relationships with clients. Here are some red flags that could signal the need for supervision:

- Having a good number of clients who seem "difficult" or controlling
- Having a lot of clients who challenge your boundaries
- Making friends with clients more than once in a blue moon
- Realizing that you take on the issues, feelings, or energy of a client in a way that depletes you
- Often feeling sexually attracted to clients
- Frequently feeling drained or exhausted at the end of the day
- Often feeling bored with your work
- Any negative feelings about clients that persist

The Power of Groups

Some practitioners prefer getting together with colleagues, either with or without a leader or consultant, to share their experiences and knowledge. Some believe that support from colleagues is a must in a profession that is so minimally recognized and acknowledged in the culture. Also, because of the element of touch, somatic practitioners face unique issues that may be understood best by their colleagues.

Many of us have little contact or serious discussion with other manual therapists. Even if we work around other massage therapists, we don't always take the time for serious discussion. I have given workshops in which bodyworkers start a question with "Maybe I'm the only one this happens to. . ." and then relate a situation that is commonly experienced by practitioners. It helps to have the reassurance that others are dealing with the same dilemmas.

People who stay with this work over the long haul are usually part of a strong group or community of colleagues that support and educate each other.

It also helps to have the validation of talking with a respected colleague or a group of colleagues when you are learning how to set boundaries and limits with your clients. Getting outside support and ideas is fortification for dealing with manipulative or hard-to-handle clients.

Especially in the first years of your practice, you may not know enough to know when you are in over your head or when what a client needs is beyond the scope of your methods or beyond your expertise. You might not fully trust your intuition or recognize a red flag.

Getting together with colleagues in an open, honest, and non-judgmental environment can be comforting, confidence building, and a boon to your practice. People who stay with this work over the long haul are usually part of a strong group or community of colleagues that support and educate each other.

Group Supervision

Less expensive than individual supervision, group supervision is great for dealing with isolation. It's also a good way for inexperienced practitioners to learn the common client-relationship issues of this work and gather ideas about the ways others deal with problems that are shared by all practitioners. As with peer support groups, hearing the struggles of others in the group can help you see that you're not alone or unique in the kind of dilemmas that you have. The difference between a peer support group and group supervision is that a supervision group is led by a supervisor and there is usually a fee for attending.

A massage therapist from Seattle praises her supervision group:

➤ *My supervision group has been getting together for a year, meeting every 3 weeks. We alternate meeting with just each other and meeting with a supervisor. Being in the group is helping me move to a place that is healthier with my client relations. For instance, I've learned that I was brought up to see my value as a person as how "helpful" and "selfless" I could be. Now I don't work so hard and long on a client that my thumbs are aching, as I used to. I won't take one more client that will be too taxing for my body or mind. I don't take responsibility for clients' healing. I empower them in their healing process. My relationships with my clients feel cleaner with less hidden agendas. And I'm making more money!*

I actually went into supervision to learn how to run my business better and make more money. But what was most helpful was that I learned about my boundary problems during the course of being in the group. It's ironic that my initial goals are being met in an entirely roundabout way!

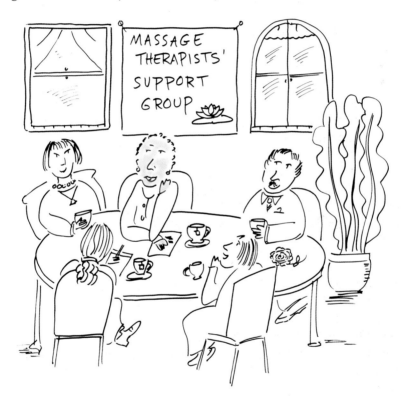

Peer Support Groups

It is possible to meet as a group of practitioners to discuss common issues without a supervisor. Peer groups are not supervised by any of the members and have different benefits than groups that include supervision. Nan Narboe, clinical social worker and boundaries expert, says:

➤ *There are things that only your peers will tell you and that you can only hear from your peers. For instance, if our supervisor praises the way we responded to a difficult client, we may assume she's "just being nice." If we hear the same praise from our peers, we tend to believe it. There are times, however, when individual supervision is best. There are things that only your supervisor will tell you and that you can only hear from your supervisor, such as where your blind spots are.*

Peer groups are an excellent and inexpensive way to get support and learn from others. Groups may also want to hire a consultant to work with them occasionally on a specific issue or for a specific purpose.

Jack Blackburn, LMP, certified Trager practitioner, registered counselor, and supervisor for bodyworkers, reinforces the need for meeting with colleagues: "The main reason practitioners burn out isn't because they work too hard or take too much responsibility for their clients. It's because they don't have a place to talk with other massage therapists and bodyworkers about what happens in their practices." In peer groups, practitioners can learn how to support each other's learning by using active listening and other techniques to help each other understand their relationships with clients.

Benefits of Supervision and Consultation

Whether you work with a group or individually, here are some of the reasons that consultations and supervision about client–practitioner dynamics are invaluable to both inexperienced and seasoned practitioners.

Identifying Blind Spots

We all have less-than-positive ways of interacting that we tend to put out of our awareness—ways that we might unconsciously hurt clients, ways that we might overstep boundaries. We need feedback from someone who has the skill and willingness to tell us what we do not see about ourselves. Our teachers don't always do this, nor do all friends, partners, or spouses. We like to think of ourselves as always caring, and it can be painful to have someone, even diplomatically, point out ways we might be insensitive to others. But how else are we going to learn?

Ethics consultant Daphne Chellos says it straight out:

➤ *Supervision is a preventive measure against abusing clients. Abuse can be unintentional as well as intentional, subtle as well as blatant. As humans, all of us can be "victims" and all of us can be "aggressors." Our tendency is to remember violations against us and to either forget or ignore our aggressive acts. This blind spot exists as well in therapeutic relationships. A competent supervisor will notice when a therapist is being inappropriate or abusive, no matter how subtly or unintentionally, and bring it to the therapist's attention. (Chellos D. Supervision in bodywork: borrowing a model from psychotherapy. Massage Ther J. 1991;Winter:15.)*

"Abuse" may seem like a strong word. It is used here to mean anything a practitioner does that could, even in a minor way, take advantage of or wound a client—from an insensitive remark about the client's body to overcharging for services.

Keeping Confidentiality

Clients tell us their secrets. Even if they don't tell us, we might guess. Perhaps we realize how frightened that successful, confident-looking businessman actually is because we see the tension in his body. Maybe we sense the underlying sadness of the vivacious woman who tries so hard to be upbeat. Clients confide in us about their private lives and concerns, but as professionals, we're not allowed to talk about our clients with our colleagues, friends, or families, and we're certainly not allowed to divulge anything they say. As Trager instructor Amrita Daigle says, "If we don't have someone who we can talk with in professional confidence, we will tend to gossip about our clients." It can become a burden to carry all that pain, all those secrets. Having a supervisor who is also bound by rules of confidentiality gives us a way to share that burden.

Easing Guilt

I've talked with many practitioners who feel ashamed of an instance when they used poor judgment or went outside ethical boundaries. Sometimes no harm was done to the client, and sometimes the practitioner couldn't have foreseen the problem. However, these moments weigh on practitioners who strive to be ethical. Talking with a trusted supervisor or consultant helps put those mistakes in perspective. A good supervisor or consultant will hear our mistakes and errors without making us feel ashamed or incompetent.

Recognizing Prejudice

How do we really feel about working with people of other races, gays and lesbians, overweight people, the chronically ill, racists, Orthodox Jews, Hindus, Muslims, and born-again Christians—just to name a few groups? What about people who voted for the candidate we campaigned against? Or sexist men, pampered women, angry feminists? Do any of these types of people make our hearts snap shut? Everyone makes prejudgments to some degree. Consultation and supervision help us recognize these prejudgments so that we can get beyond our negative feelings and learn to either care about the client or refer the client to someone else.

Getting Help with Mentally Ill Clients

We will probably encounter emotionally disturbed people in our practices, and they will respond to us and our work differently than will other clients. We may be baffled by their behavior or be insensitive to their fears. Or we may not know how to take care of ourselves when we are working with them. A consultant trained in psychological dynamics is a valuable resource for helping us identify and figure out what to do with clients who may be mentally ill.

Clients with mental illness can make complaints or feel harmed even when practitioners are ethical and careful. As caring practitioners, we may want to help a client who appears to be floundering. Yet some people who are mentally ill can exhibit extreme helplessness on the one hand and rage on the other. We may be ill-fatedly drawn to try to rescue a seemingly helpless client, only to wind up as the recipient of that person's anger. For our own protection, we need help identifying mental illness.

Although it is not our place to make a specific diagnosis, we do want to know whether a client is mentally ill for his or her protection as well as our own. For example, people with a mental illness generally don't have the interior strength to weather a process that can strip away defenses, such as emotionally-oriented work. Ordinary folks seek out that kind of work to experience a deeper part of themselves. For disturbed people, who may feel blank or chaotic behind their social exterior, such work can be uncomfortable and disorienting. An experienced consultant or supervisor can help us identify signs of mental illness and judge whether our work will be beneficial to the prospective client. Of course, if the client is being treated by a mental health professional, we should obtain written permission from the client to speak with the other professional to make sure our work will be helpful to the client.

Supporting Our Intuition

Many manual therapists use their intuition to understand how best to work with clients. Intuition is a useful gift, but sometimes it fails us. Sometimes clients slip beneath the radar of our intuition, or we need more information to be able to understand them. We may misread them and fail to offer the kind of support they need. A consultant or supervisor could help us see the reasons we didn't understand the client and educate us about how best to use our intuitive side.

And the #1 Reason for Getting Consultation or Supervision

Perhaps it's a little late to say this, but good boundaries can't be entirely learned from reading a book. We have to experience them. We need to experience the safety of working with someone who is clear and careful with boundaries. We have to get the solid feeling of good boundaries inside us.

A book can give us an idea of why it's important to be professional, but we can't learn it all from a book. Some may have had a teacher along the way who was careless or uneducated about relationship issues, and we need a remedial experience. If we aspire to a high level of professionalism, we need the good modeling that a compassionate professional trained in transference and countertransference can provide.

Finding Help and Support

For manual therapists, getting help with the relationship aspect of our work and coming together to support each other are still new concepts. Certainly, practitioners get together informally with friends who are also bodyworkers to encourage each other and talk about common issues. However, more organized ways of meeting together are still not that widely practiced. But casual sharing, aside from the possibility of leading to violations of confidentiality, doesn't always offer the depth of support and insight that we need. Fortunately, practitioners can now find and create other ways to enrich their professional lives.

Choosing a Consultant or Supervisor

Because getting consultations and supervision for the relationship issues of this work is a fairly new idea, you will have to be creative in finding someone with whom to work. The practitioner you choose should be someone who is trained in psychological dynamics and understands and appreciates bodywork and massage. A psychiatric social worker, psychologist, or other mental health professional who has never experienced bodywork may not be able to understand the intimacy of the work and the problems involved. Your consultant or supervisor should also respect the profession and be aware that manual therapists perform a valuable service for the community.

You can also work with a bodyworker or massage therapist who has training and experience in relationship dynamics. Although that would be ideal, few manual practitioners have such training.

No set way exists to find someone who will suit you. You can ask others for the names of good psychotherapists in your community and see if they would be interested in working with you. They have to understand that you don't want personal counseling, and they need to know the difference between consulting about work issues and doing psychotherapy. Not all psychotherapists have the experience or the inclination to do this kind of consulting.

Because you are hoping to learn more about good relationship boundaries, it should be obvious that your consultant or supervisor needs to be someone with whom you don't have another relationship.

Keep in mind that because the consultant or supervisor doesn't need to see your hands-on work, supervision and consultation can occur by phone. If you live in

You want some-one who gives you the feeling that you have a new ally, that you have someone in your corner.

a small town, you may choose to have telephone appointments with an out-of-town consultant who does not know your clients.

When you are trying out a supervisor or consultant, you want to notice if this is someone who helps you trust your own intuition, who can suggest new choices without making you feel judged, who is enthusiastic about your work, and who helps you feel more confident. You want someone who gives you the feeling that you have a new ally, that you have someone in your corner.

Forming a Peer Group

While in school, many students form close bonds with other students but do not keep in touch once they have graduated. Once out in their practices, massage therapists and bodyworkers don't always have an awareness of how crucial it is to their professional health to stay in touch with colleagues.

To start a group, you have to round up some colleagues who would like to get together regularly to share experiences. An ideal number would be between 4 and 12 participants. It's a good idea to ask members to commit to meeting on a regular schedule for a certain length of time—perhaps once or twice a month for at least six meetings—to give the group a chance to gel.

Groups need to adhere to rules of confidentiality in agreeing not to talk outside the group about what other members say there. Also, members should agree to make every effort to disguise the identity of clients they are discussing.

It's a good idea if group members agree to other ground rules as well, such as not offering advice unless they are asked to or not interrupting others. Care should be taken to give each member a chance to bring their issues to the group. Although a small amount of venting can be useful, groups shouldn't be allowed to deteriorate into gripe sessions.

It's important that groups state their intentions clearly from the beginning, for instance, that they're interested in learning from each other and wanting to grow as professionals.

One important consideration may be that you belong to, or form, a group of like-minded individuals . . . people who have similar practices. For example, if you are an evidence-informed practitioner of massage, you may not feel comfortable in a room full of people who practice energy work, and vice versa.

A Word about Mentoring

With mentoring, you make an agreement with a more experienced colleague that she or he will be available to answer your questions. It can be an informal arrangement and is often unpaid. It may be as simple as, "Let me take you to lunch and get the benefit of your years as a bodyworker." Everyone graduating from manual therapy training needs mentors. It should be a given that we all need help and support to start a practice.

Mentoring usually addresses less complex issues than supervision does. It's good for business-building and practice-building kinds of questions, such as the value of using an answering service or the pros and cons of working out of your home.

A mentor can be any practitioner you respect, whose work is similar to yours and who is willing to meet with you to share his or her experiences.

These days, it's even possible to find excellent mentoring on an online forum for massage therapists or bodyworkers. On such forums, there are hundreds of massage therapists and bodyworkers with varying levels of experience. Participants can ask questions that they would ask a mentor and receive a wide range of advice. The obvious disadvantage of this method is that there isn't the face-to-face relationship that can provide ongoing encouragement and support, and you don't necessarily know the qualifications of the people responding.

Taking Care of Ourselves

To forestall burnout, somatic practitioners need to learn how to take good care of themselves, which means getting help from others. Sharing with someone else about what really goes on in our offices, what pushes our buttons, and when our hearts get shut down is crucial to the health of our practices.

The work we do is complex and demanding. Consultations, supervision, peer support, and mentoring can take away the isolation and depletion that can kill our interest in our work. Our professional lives are more rewarding when we find ways to keep our interest alive and be kinder to ourselves.

Questions for Reflection

1. If you are a student, what steps can you take when you finish your training to make sure you have the support and information you need? If you are already practicing, do you have enough support to keep you excited and encouraged about your work? Do you have any resources to help you sort out the therapeutic relationship aspect of your work? What steps could you take to make sure you have enough support and resources?

2. How do you feel about the idea of going to someone for supervision or consultation? What would be the pros and cons for you personally?

3. Are there areas where you could benefit from help—for instance, setting limits, working with women who have been sexually abused, or knowing how to work with an emotionally-fragile client? What are the areas that

are the most challenging for you? What can you do to help you feel more confident about these areas?

4. If you are already practicing, can you think of a time when a problem with a client would have gone much smoothly if you had had outside professional help with it? How would you handle that situation now?

---

thePoint® To learn more about the concepts discussed in this chapter, visit http://thePoint .lww.com/Allen-McIntosh4e

American Massage Therapy Association Code of Ethics

This Code of Ethics is a summary statement of the standards by which massage therapists agree to conduct their practices and is a declaration of the general principles of acceptable, ethical, professional behavior.

Massage therapists/practitioners shall:

1. Demonstrate commitment to provide the highest quality massage therapy/bodywork to those who seek their professional service.
2. Acknowledge the inherent worth and individuality of each person by not discriminating or behaving in any prejudicial manner with clients and/or colleagues.
3. Demonstrate professional excellence through regular self-assessment of strengths, limitations, and effectiveness by continued education and training.
4. Acknowledge the confidential nature of the professional relationship with clients and respect each client's right to privacy.
5. Project a professional image and uphold the highest standards of professionalism.
6. Accept responsibility to do no harm to the physical, mental and emotional well-being of self, clients, and associates.

AMTA goes further by spelling out the Rules of Ethics:

Massage therapists/practitioners shall do the following:

1. Conduct all business and professional activities within their scope of practice and all applicable legal and regulatory requirements.
2. Refrain from engaging in any sexual conduct or sexual activities involving their clients in the course of a massage therapy session.

3. Be truthful in advertising and marketing, and refrain from misrepresenting his or her services, charges for services, credentials, training, experience, ability, or results.

4. Refrain from using AMTA membership, including the AMTA name, logo or other intellectual property, or the member's position, in any way that is unauthorized, improper, or misleading.

5. Refrain from engaging in any activity that would violate confidentiality commitments and/or proprietary rights of AMTA or any other person or organization.

Appendix B

Associated Bodywork and Massage Professionals Code of Ethics

As a member of Associated Bodywork and Massage Professionals (ABMP), I pledge my commitment to the highest principles of the massage and bodywork profession as outlined here:

1. Commitment to High-Quality Care

I will serve the best interests of my clients at all times and provide the highest quality of bodywork and service possible. I recognize that the obligation for building and maintaining an effective, healthy, and safe therapeutic relationship with my clients is my responsibility.

2. Commitment to Do No Harm

I will conduct a thorough health history intake process for each client and evaluate the health history to rule out contraindications or determine appropriate session adaptations. If I see signs of, or suspect, an undiagnosed condition that massage may be inappropriate for, I will refer that client to a physician or other qualified health-care professional and delay the massage session until approval from the physician has been granted. I understand the importance of ethical touch and therapeutic intent and will conduct sessions with the sole objective of benefitting the client.

3. Commitment to Honest Representation of Qualifications

I will not work outside the commonly accepted scope of practice for massage therapists and bodywork professionals. I will adhere to my state's scope of practice guidelines (when applicable). I will only provide treatments and techniques for which I am fully trained and hold credible credentials. I will carefully evaluate the needs of each client and refer the client to another provider if the client requires work beyond my capabilities, or beyond the capacity of massage and bodywork. I will not use the trademarks and symbols associated with a particular system or group without authentic affiliation. I will acknowledge the limitations of massage

249

and bodywork by refraining from exaggerating the benefits of massage therapy and related services throughout my marketing.

4. Commitment to Uphold the Inherent Worth of All Individuals

I will demonstrate compassion, respect, and tolerance for others. I will seek to decrease discrimination, misunderstandings, and prejudice. I understand there are situations when it is appropriate to decline service to a client because it is in the best interests of a client's health, or for my personal safety, but I will not refuse service to any client based on disability, ethnicity, gender, marital status, physical build, or sexual orientation; religious, national, or political affiliation; social or economic status.

5. Commitment to Respect Client Dignity and Basic Rights

I will demonstrate my respect for the dignity and rights of all individuals by providing a clean, comfortable, and safe environment for sessions, using appropriate and skilled draping procedures, giving the clients recourse in the event of dissatisfaction with treatment, and upholding the integrity of the therapeutic relationship.

6. Commitment to Informed Consent

I will recognize a client's right to determine what happens to his or her body. I understand that a client may suffer emotional and physical harm if a therapist fails to listen to the client and imposes his or her own beliefs on a situation. I will fully inform my clients of choices relating to their care, and disclose policies and limitations that may affect their care. I will not provide massage without obtaining a client's informed consent (or that of the guardian or advocate for the client) to the session plan.

7. Commitment to Confidentiality

I will keep client communication and information confidential and will not share client information without the client's written consent, within the limits of the law. I will ensure every effort is made to respect a client's right to privacy and provide an environment where personal health-related details cannot be overheard or seen by others.

8. Commitment to Personal and Professional Boundaries

I will refrain from and prevent behaviors that may be considered sexual in my massage practice and uphold the highest professional standards in order to desexualize massage. I will not date a client, engage in sexual intercourse with a client, or allow any level of sexual impropriety (behavior or language) from clients or myself. I understand that sexual impropriety may lead to sexual harassment charges, the loss of my massage credentials, lawsuits for personal damages, criminal charges, fines, attorney's fees, court costs, and jail time.

9. Commitment to Honesty in Business

I will know and follow good business practices with regard to record keeping, regulation compliance, and tax law. I will set fair fees and practice honesty throughout my marketing materials. I will not accept gifts, compensation, or other benefits intended to influence a decision related to a client. If I use the Associated Bodywork & Massage Professionals logo, I promise to do so appropriately to establish my credibility and market my practice.

10. Commitment to Professionalism

I will maintain clear and honest communication with clients and colleagues. I will not use recreational drugs or alcohol before or during massage sessions. I will project a professional image with respect to my behavior and personal appearance in keeping with the highest standards of the massage profession. I will not actively seek to take someone else's clients, disrespect a client or colleague, or willingly malign another therapist or other allied professional. I will actively strive to positively promote the massage and bodywork profession by committing to self-development and continually building my professional skills.

Appendix C

Related Readings

Benjamin BE, Sohnen-Moe CM. The Ethics of Touch: The Practitioner's Guide to Creating a Professional, Safe, and Enduring Practice. Tucson, AZ: Sohnen-Moe Associates, 2013.

Benjamin P. Professional Foundations for Massage Therapists. Upper Saddle River, NJ: Prentice Hall, 2008.

Borysenko J. Minding the Body, Mending the Mind. Boston, MA: Da Capo Press, 2007.

Fanning P, McKay M, Davis M. Messages: The Communication Skills Book, 3rd ed. Oakland, CA: New Harbinger Publications, 2009.

Ford CW. Compassionate Touch: The Body's Role in Emotional Healing and Recovery, 2nd ed. Berkeley, CA: North Atlantic Books, 1999.

Frank JD, Frank JB. Persuasion and Healing. Baltimore, MD: Johns Hopkins University Press, 1993.

Giroud B. Ethics and Professionalism for Massage Therapists and Bodyworkers. Upper Saddle River, NJ: Pearson, 2013.

Greene E, Goodrich-Dunn B. The Psychology of the Body, 2nd ed. Baltimore, MD: Lippincott, Williams & Wilkins, 2013.

Herman JL. Trauma and Recovery: The Aftermath of Violence—From Domestic Abuse to Political Terror. New York, NY: Basic Books, 2015.

Naparstek B. Invisible Heroes: Survivors of Trauma and How They Heal. New York, NY: Bantam, 2004.

Taylor K. The Ethics of Caring: Honoring the Web of Life in Our Professional Healing Relationships. Santa Cruz, CA: Hanford Mead, 1995.

Thompson DL. Hands Heal: Communication, Documentation, and Insurance Billing for Manual Therapists, 4th ed. Baltimore, MD: Lippincott Williams & Wilkins, 2011.

Yardley-Nohr T. Ethics for Massage Therapists. Baltimore, MD: Lippincott Williams & Wilkins, 2007.

Altered state: A state of consciousness in which we are more deeply relaxed, less aware of our thinking minds, and more open and vulnerable than we are in our day-to-day functioning.

Bartering: Used here to mean exchanging a manual therapy session for goods or services other than another manual therapy session.

Boundaries: In this context, a boundary is like a protective circle around the professional relationship that separates what is appropriate between practitioner and client from what is not. Keeping appropriate boundaries includes such behavior as not engaging a client in another kind of relationship, such as a social one, and honoring what is appropriate within the professional relationship, such as confidentiality.

Consultation: A meeting with a professional trained in psychological dynamics to obtain advice and insight about a particular client or issue.

Contract: An agreement between practitioner and client that is often implied rather than explicit about what each will or will not do. An ethical contract must be within the bounds of the practitioner's training and the ethical standards of her or his profession. The client agrees to give specific fees, goods, or services in return and agrees to be respectful of the practitioner's guidelines for appropriate behavior.

Countertransference: When a practitioner allows unresolved feelings and personal issues to influence his relationship with a client.

Dual relationships: Having a relationship with a client other than the contractual therapeutic one, such as having a client who is also a friend, family member, or business associate.

Emotionally-oriented bodywork: Manual therapy that is based on the idea that physical tension and restriction are related to unconscious patterns of holding that the client has adopted, often early in life, to cope with his or her emotional environment. The practitioner facilitates the client in releasing these tension patterns for the greater emotional and physical well-being of the client. Also called, *psychologically-oriented bodywork*.

Framework: The logistics by which practitioners define themselves as professional and create a safe atmosphere for clients. Framework includes the ways that we present ourselves in advertising, the preparation of the physical setting, policies on fees and time, and such ground rules as keeping the focus on the client.

Informed consent: The client's authorization for services to be performed by the practitioner. The client or the client's guardian must be fully advised of what the service will entail and its benefits and any contraindications and must be competent to give consent.

Manual therapists: Trained professionals who touch the physical or energetic body of the client using a method of movement to affect the body of a client for the purpose of facilitating awareness, health, and well-being. The term as used here is interchangeable with *somatic practitioners* and includes massage therapists, bodyworkers, movement educators, practitioners of Eastern methods, and practitioners who work primarily with energy fields.

Mentor: A trusted colleague who provides guidance and education. Mentors are usually helpful in advising on both the details of establishing oneself as a professional and the broader general aspects of taking on a professional role or of taking on the role of a particular kind of bodywork or massage practitioner.

Peer group: A group of colleagues who meet regularly to discuss common issues related to their professional lives, to share information and strategies, and to receive emotional support.

Posttraumatic stress disorder (PTSD): A type of anxiety disorder that can develop after experiencing a very traumatic or life-threatening event. It can cause flashbacks; sleep problems; nightmares; hypervigilance; feelings of isolation, guilt, and paranoia; and sometimes panic attacks.

Power differential: A concept used to describe a professional relationship where one person is viewed to have more knowledge and authority than the other, such as the client–therapist relationship.

Professional therapeutic relationship: A relationship between client and practitioner that is focused on the well-being of the client and is contractual.

Right of refusal: The entitlement of both the client and the practitioner to end a session or to decline to receive or give a particular kind of manipulation or technique.

Role-playing: Usually a structured exercise in which students or colleagues take a role—for instance, as client or practitioner—and act out a specific situation as a way of becoming more comfortable with handling the situation in real life.

Scope of practice: The traditional knowledge base and standard practices of the profession.

Sliding scale: Using a sliding scale to determine fees means that you offer a range of fees based on the client's income. For instance, someone who has a low salary would pay your lowest rate of $40 per hour and a wealthier person would pay your standard rate of $90 an hour, with gradations in between.

Supervision: An ongoing arrangement made with a professional trained in psychological dynamics for help with the relationship aspects of a practitioner's work. Supervision includes clarifying the client's transference issues and the practitioner's countertransference issues, suggesting effective interventions and identifying the practitioner's vulnerabilities and areas of strength.

Therapeutic contract: An agreement between practitioner and client that is often implied rather than being explicit about what each will or will not do. An ethical contract must be within the bounds of the practitioner's training and the ethical standards of his or her profession. The client agrees to give specific fees, goods, or services in return and agrees to be respectful of the practitioner's guidelines for appropriate behavior.

Therapeutic relationship: A relationship between client and practitioner that is focused on the well-being of the client.

Trade: Exchanging a manual therapy session for a manual therapy session with a colleague.

Transference: When a client unconsciously projects (transfers) unresolved feelings, needs, and issues—usually from childhood and usually related to parent or other authority figures—onto a practitioner.